PROFESSIONAL NURSE SERIES

Infection Control made Easy

A Hospital Guide for Health Professionals

Ansie Minnaar

Series editor: Nelouise Geyer

JUTA

Infection Control made Easy

© Juta and Co Ltd, 2008
Mercury Crescent, Hillstar
Wetton, 7780
Cape Town, South Africa

ISBN 978 0 7021 7720 0

Project manager: Marlinee Chetty
Editor: Danya Ristic
Proofreading and indexing: Ethné Clarke
Cover design: Alexander Kornonov of Studio Art
Design and typeset in 11/13 pt Berkley Oldstyle Book by Mckore Graphics
Printed and bound in the Republic of South Africa by Mills Litho, Maitland, CapeTown

Contents

How to use this book viii

Chapter One: Introduction and history of infection control 1
Introduction 3
The history of infection control 3
Factors contributing to the emergence of infectious diseases 5
Quality control standards for infection control 6
Precautions 7
Case study 9
Tips for nurses 9
Conclusion 10
Self-assessment 11
Further reading and web resources 11

Chapter Two: Hand-washing in health care organisations 12
Introduction 14
Transmission of pathogens 14
Factors influencing adherence to hand hygiene practices 15
Hand hygiene guidelines 17
Hand hygiene in the case of specific organisms 19
Significant aspects of hand-washing compliance 20
Case study 23
Tips for nurses 23
Precautions 24
Conclusion 24
Self-assessment 24
Further reading and web resources 25

Chapter Three: Disinfection and sterilisation 26
Introduction 28
Procedure for terminal cleaning 28
Management of blood spills and infectious spills 29
Disinfection of items used in hospital 29
Case study 30
Tips for nurses 33
Precautions 33
Conclusion 34

Self-assessment..34
Further reading and web resources 34

Chapter Four: Environmental aspects of the prevention of nosocomial infection...**35**
Introduction...37
The hospital environment and specific interventions 38
Surveillance system 40
Principles of infection control 40
Infection control assessment guide......................................41
Management of an outbreak..42
Case study...43
Tips for nurses 44
Precautions...44
Conclusion..44
Self-assessment...44
Further reading and web resources 44

Chapter Five: Critical issues in infection control **45**
Introduction...47
Urinary tract infection (catheter-associated) 48
Surgical site infection 49
Bloodstream infection (IV device-associated)......................54
Pneumonia (ventilator-associated) 57
Case study...58
Tips for nurses 58
Precautions...59
Conclusion..60
Self-assessment...60
Further reading and web resources 60

Chapter Six: African haemorrhagic fevers.......................**61**
Introduction...62
Arenaviridae – Lassa fever 63
Bunyaviridae (phlebovirus) – Rift Valley fever....................64
Bunyaviridae (nairovirus) – Congo-Crimea 65
Filoviridae filovirus – Ebola and Marburg fever..................66
Flavivirus – Yellow fever...67
Case study...67
Tips for nurses 70

Precautions 70
Conclusion 70
Self-assessment 70
Further reading and web resources 71

Chapter Seven: Emerging infections 72
Introduction 74
Avian flu 74
Severe acute respiratory syndrome 75
Multiple drug-resistant TB and extremely drug-resistant TB 76
HIV and Aids 77
Case study 79
Tips for nurses 79
Precautions 79
Conclusion 79
Self-assessment 80
Further reading and web resources 80

Conclusion 81

References 82

Index 85

How to use this book

This publication forms part of a series for the continuous professional development of professional nurses. The overall goal of this series is to provide an integrated approach to the topic under discussion. Each book in the series can be used by individuals or groups or as an education and training resource by nursing education institutions for learning experiences on the topic addressed.

An author who has knowledge and expertise in the particular subject has prepared each publication. It is hoped that this book will meet your learning and development needs by presenting the content in an easily accessible and user-friendly way that will facilitate learning.

Each publication addresses a specific topic in nursing, and is divided into separate chapters. The introduction includes:
- learning outcomes that you could expect to achieve after completing the course,
- the learning that is assumed to be in place, and
- key ethical and legislative considerations of which the nurse should take cognisance.

Each chapter contains:
- information and examples relating to the topic,
- learning activities with questions that allow you to apply the information in your own context,
- case study(ies) relating to the content of the chapter, and
- notes containing tips and precautions for your information, where applicable.

A separate answer guide, containing main points for consideration, is included at the back of this book.

Enjoy the learning experience!

Nelouise Geyer
Series editor
January 2008

CHAPTER ONE

Introduction and history of infection control

Learning outcomes

Upon completion of this chapter, you should be able to:

- discuss the history of infection control
- identify the precaution methods and describe how and when each one applies.

Learning assumed to be in place

To gain the most benefit from this chapter, you should already have the following knowledge and skills:

- An understanding of infectious diseases and how they spread in communities and hospitals.
- The ability to read a microbiology report on a patient with an infectious disease.

Key ethical considerations

- Health care workers and nursing staff have the obligation to use their skills and knowledge to prevent nosocomial infections.
- Health care workers and nurses must identify and implement precautions in cases of infected patients.
- Nurses are obliged to prevent any harm or infection to patients in all circumstances.

Key legislative considerations

- All health care workers are governed by Acts and regulations, such as the *National Health Act (61 of 2003)*.
- Nurses have a legal obligation to comply with the Acts regulating their practice as professional nurses, for example the *Nursing Act, 2005 (Act 33 of 2005)*.
- The *Constitution of the Republic of South Africa (Act 108 of 1996, Section 24)*.
- The *Occupational Health and Safety Act (85 of 1993, Section 8(1))*.
- *Government Notice R1390, 27 December 2001, Section 43* (HBA Regulations).
- The *Environmental Conservation Act (73 of 1989)*.

Important terms

- Nosocomial infection, or hospital-acquired infection (HAI), is defined as any infection that a person develops as a result of treatment in hospital.
- Precautions entail isolating a patient from other patients and staff either because their condition renders them at risk of infection to others or because they themselves are potentially a source of infection.
- Standard precautions imply the washing of hands after touching blood, bodily fluids, secretions, excretions and contaminated items, regardless of wearing gloves.
- An airborne precaution involves placing the patient in a private room with negative air pressure.
- Droplet precautions entail placing the patient in a private room, if available. A mask must be worn by anyone working within a metre of the patient.
- Contact precautions consist of placing the patient in a private room, if available. A mask must be worn by anyone working within a metre of the patient. The patient is transported out of the room only when necessary. A surgical mask should be placed on the patient if possible.
- A surveillance system for health care services must provide adequate structures and resources, including staff, for successful infection control.
- A vector is an organism that transmits a particular disease or parasite from one plant or animal to another.
- A lazaretto is an isolation hospital for people with an infectious disease.

INTRODUCTION

Infection control in health services comprises a set of principles and guidelines for improving quality of care given to patients. Infection control is part of risk management in any health service. In the general population, infection control is concerned with food and water supplies, and effective waste disposal, which contribute to an increased life expectancy for community members. In health care facilities, these basic concerns also apply – health and food legislation and various control mechanisms impose obligations on hospitals and health care services to ensure a safe environment for patients and staff.

Nosocomial infections, that is, hospital-acquired infections, remain an important issue in hospitals, the cost of which is difficult to measure. Health care services must learn to see infection rates as a quality indicator for accreditation of the hospital. A robust surveillance system and infection control programmes need to be in place. The surveillance system must provide:

- adequate structures and resources, including staff, for successful infection control
- policies and standards for effective control of infections
- written programmes, effective measures for data collection, a reporting system for infection rates, and training programmes for all categories of staff on infection control (Weaving & Cooper 2006: 18).

THE HISTORY OF INFECTION CONTROL

Worldwide infectious diseases place a considerable burden on health care individuals and organisations. Infectious diseases take a greater toll on infants and young children, and disproportionately affect populations in developing countries. It is clear that we do not learn from experience when it comes to infectious diseases. As early as 3000 BC, the Egyptians saw infection as a punishment. Personal hygiene was emphasised on papyrus scrolls.

Ancient suffering is evident from various sources, for example in research done on the tissues of mummies. Drop foot was evident from polio, and Pott's disease, which affected the spine, was evident from tuberculosis (TB). Tetanus, an extremely old disease, was also found in mummies. Factors contributing to the elimination of infections were improved, and hygiene, sanitation and higher standards of socio-economic conditions facilitated the elimination of vectors. Later, during the 20th century, immunisation against infectious diseases and high standards of hygiene eliminated and controlled infections.

The Greek physician Hippocrates (370–460 BC), who coined the phrase 'Do no harm', was the first person to refer to infection control and the avoidance of harming the patient. The Greek philosopher Aristotle (384–322 BC) believed that doctors should observe diseases. During the time of the Roman civilisation, much was done to improve the health and living conditions of the people. The Romans built roads, and designed houses with underfloor heating. They also invented flushing toilets with a sewer system. Later, people with leprosy were sent outside cities to lazarettos, which can be compared to today's isolation units or isolation hospitals. This was the first separation of healthy and ill people (Larson 1989: 92–9).

The plague, or typhus virus, was first identified in the sixth century AD, and thereafter in the Middle Ages, around 1600, and later, in 1867, in America, Europe, Russia and Africa. The disease is an ongoing problem; even today, in 2007, we find plague in African countries such as Zimbabwe and Namibia. Doctors wore goggles, masks and long cloaks in the early days of the plague, which contributed to the problem, as the material harboured the fleas that carried the disease. Plague was also transported on ships, via rats.

Syphilis was known as the 'angry, aggressive disease', and during explorer Christopher Columbus's (1451–1506) sea journeys it spread around the globe. It was called 'Naples' at first, because it seemed to originate from there. Later, syphilis and gonorrhoea were seen as being one and the same disease. Anton van Leeuwenhoek (1632–1723) was the first person to look through a microscope in the 17th century and notice that the organisms looked different. Edwin Jenner (1749–1823) first attempted to inoculate humans as a protection against smallpox. During the 1700s, all sewage from Paris was allowed to drain into the Seine River, from which people also obtained their drinking water. In those days, hospitals would have about 1 000 beds and at any give time about 3 000 patients. In some places, little has changed – in South Africa today we have three babies per incubator and more than one patient per bed in our public hospitals!

British hospitals, by contrast, were cleaner, with sheets being washed once in three weeks and there being no more than one patient per bed. During the 1800s, the water in London was contaminated and the resulting cholera and typhoid killed many people. Ignaz Semmelweis (1818–1865) emphasised the washing of hands with chloredine solution (chlorhexidine) in maternity hospitals in Vienna and Italy. Puerperal sepsis was reduced once doctors began to wash their hands after performing autopsies and before delivering babies (Best & Neuhauser 2004: 233–4; Dunn 2005: 345–8).

During the Industrial Revolution, smallpox, typhoid and TB had disastrous effects. Cleaners threw urine and faeces through the windows of buildings and out onto the streets, which caused infection to spread quickly. Towards the end of the 19th century, hygiene started to improve. However, while households were kept cleaner, TB continued to pose a problem. Florence Nightingale (1820–1910) recorded hospital-based statistics, separated patients into different wards according to their diseases, and effectively conducted other epidemiological work. Louis Pasteur (1822–1895) invented the process of pasteurisation and tried to find a vaccination against anthrax. Joseph Lister (1827–1912) described antisepsis and asepsis. He promoted carbolic acid in the cleaning of hospitals, which decreased the infection rates.

Furthermore, Robert Koch (1843–1910) defended the process of disinfection in his germ theory, proposing that every disease has a cause and that viruses cannot be cultured. From Koch's (1890) postulates we know now that hospitals need surveillance systems and evidence or proof of infection control procedures and control methods, to be able to control infections.

Koch's (1890) postulates stated firstly, micro-organisms must be found in all organisms suffering from the disease, but not in healthy organisms. Secondly, micro-organisms must be isolated from a diseased organism and grown in pure culture. Thirdly, the cultured micro-organism should cause disease when introduced into a healthy organism and lastly the micro-organism must be re-isolated from the inoculated. These postulates of Koch changes over the years as the medical sciences developed and technology in the laboratories improved (Best & Neuhauser 2004: 233; Dunn 2005: 348).

Further, we know that staff in hospitals do not always comply with hand-washing procedures, old diseases still exist and antibiotics cannot solve every infection problem in modern hospitals. Crucial strategies are needed to combat infections, such as basic principles of infection control, hygiene and sanitation, anti-microbial policies, sterilisation and disinfection, hand-washing protocols and the policy of one bed per patient (Dunn 2005: 245–348).

FACTORS CONTRIBUTING TO THE EMERGENCE OF INFECTIOUS DISEASES

The following are contributing factors to general infections, which hospital staff need to consider in order to successfully control the spread of infection:

- Microbial adaptation and change, for example strains that became more virulent.
- Human susceptibility to infection.
- Climate and weather, for example heavy rains may generate breeding sites for mosquitoes and can cause malaria in sub-tropical areas.
- Changing ecosystems, for example dam-building in an area may cause vector ecology changes.
- Human demographics and behaviour, for example body-piercing and the related potential hepatitis C infection.
- Economic development and land use, for example clearing of forests can increase the mouse population and lead to outbreak of disease.
- International travel and commerce, for example the import of meat products and potentially related Creutzfeldt-Jakob and other diseases.
- Technology and industry, for example the treatment of infected chickens with fluoroquinolones and the resistance of humans to other organisms.
- Breakdown of public health measures, for example vector control and outbreak of disease.
- Poverty and social inequality, for example people becoming infected as a result of eating animals that have died from a disease.
- The disruption of public services and control measures, caused, for example,

by war and civil unrest, and by overcrowding, which can result in the spread of infectious diseases.
- Lack of political will in cases of severe acute respiratory syndrome (SARS) and other emerging diseases.
- The intent to cause harm in biological warfare and the possibility that biological weapons are related to the spread of bacillus (Lashley 2006: 4).

QUALITY CONTROL STANDARDS FOR INFECTION CONTROL

Infection control is everyone's business, not simply the role of a few specialists. Infection control must be mandated at the highest level of management in hospitals. Moreover, it must be the responsibility of the hospital board, with clear lines of accountability at hospital board level. Each hospital must have an infection control committee and an infection control team that have an annual programme providing clear objectives and priorities for surveillance and monitoring of infections. The infection control policy must reflect current guidelines on infection control, as well as legislative issues and evidence of annual audits thereof. Specialist microbiologists must support the infection control team, which should present annual and monthly reports. All health care staff, including support staff, must receive training in infection control (Weaving & Cooper 2006: 18–19).

Infection control actions

In order for infection control to be effective and efficient, the following actions must be in place in health services:

Conducting surveillance and investigation

This involves mandatory surveillance of:
- methicillin-resistant *Staphylococcus aureus* (MRSA) and *Clostridium difficile*
- surgical site infections
- serious infection-related incidents
- infections arising after hospital discharge.

Moreover, root cause analysis of food-processing systems should be done to establish the problem areas. Information should be provided to clinical teams about their infection rates. Serious outbreaks must be reported to hospital management and the Department of Health.

Reducing the infection risks of medical devices

The best-practice guidelines for use of urinary tract catheters, intravenous cannulae and other devices, and the decontamination of re-useable devices, must be implemented. Unit managers must work with infection control officers regarding adequate isolation facilities and procedures for dealing with various micro-organisms.

High standards of cleaning of equipment and of the environment must be in place, and all parties need to be on board with the latest developments. Infection control teams must be involved in the planning of hospitals and health care facilities in order to ensure the minimum risk for nosocomial infections. Proper waste and pest control needs to be in place to prevent the spread of disease.

Practising high standards of hygiene in the clinical setting

Clinical teams must demonstrate high levels of compliance with the hand-washing policy and other standard infection control precautions, all of which should frequently be measured. Awareness programmes must also be in place. Induction programmes on infection control for all staff, including agency and locums, to ensure high standards of care must always be given to patients without infection risks. Infection control must be considered part of staff development for every staff member in a health service. Each member must be up to date with immunisation prescriptions and guidelines.

Using antibiotics prudently

Antibiotics must be used prudently and according to standards set by the Department of Health and hospital boards.

Providing effective management and organisation

Heads of clinical units must ensure that infection control forms a core part of clinical governance and patient safety, and promotes low levels of infection at all times. The organisation will designate an officer for infection control, which could comprise a medical officer and a nursing professional. Accreditation teams will give high priority to the assessment of performance in reducing infections, and will pay attention to infection control policy and implementation.

Conducting research and development

A national research strategy should be formulated to focus on infection control. A rapid review process for the assessment of new products for usage in hospitals must be put in place (Weaving & Cooper 2006: 20).

PRECAUTIONS

There are specified precautions for infection control for general and specific circumstances in health services to protect every patient and staff member. Staff should acquaint themselves with these precautions so that they can safeguard against nosocomial infections. There are different levels of precautions:

- Standard precautions, which prevail as the basic level of infection control in the treatment of every patient, regardless of their diagnosis or infectious status.
- Airborne precautions in specific cases, such as TB.

- Droplet precautions in the case of infections spread by large particle droplets, such as *Neisseria meningitides*, pertussis, streptococcal pharyngitis, multi-drug-resistant *Streptococcus pneumoniae*, influenza, measles, mumps and rubella.
- Contact precautions, as most of the nosocomial infections are spread along this route, either by direct or indirect contact. Examples of micro-organisms spread by contact include *Staphylococcus aureus* (*S. aureus*), *Clostridium difficile* (*C. difficile*) and herpes simplex.

Standard precautions

- Wash hands after touching blood, bodily fluids, secretions, excretions and contaminated items, regardless of wearing gloves. Wash hands immediately after gloves are removed, between patient contacts, and whenever indicated to prevent transfer of micro-organisms to other patients. Use plain soap for routine hand-washing and an anti-microbial agent in specific circumstances.
- Wear clean, non-sterile gloves when touching blood, bodily fluids, excretions and secretions, contaminated items, mucous membranes and non-intact skin. Change gloves and wash hands between patients and tasks.
- Wear a mask, eye protection or face shield during procedures and care activities that are likely to generate sprays of blood or bodily fluids. Use a gown as part of personal protection and to protect the skin. Prevent soiling of clothes by wearing an additional plastic apron over the gown.
- Ensure that patient care equipment that is soiled with blood, bodily fluids, secretions or excretions is handled carefully and with gloves to prevent transfer of micro-organisms. Clean appropriately.
- Use adequate environmental controls to ensure that routine care, cleaning and disinfection procedures are followed. All hospital staff must be trained regarding the correct procedures.
- Handle the transportation and processing of linen soiled with blood, bodily fluids, excretions or secretions in a manner that prevents exposures and contamination of clothing and transfer of organisms.
- Take preventative measures when using needles, sharps and scalpels, and place them in the appropriate containers.

Airborne precautions

- Place the patient in a private room with negative air pressure.
- Use respiratory protection when entering the room of a patient with known suspected TB, namely, a mask (N-95 respirator).
- Transport the patient out of the room only when necessary, and place a surgical mask on the patient if possible.
- Consult infection control for preventative strategies.

Droplet precautions

- Use a private room, if available. Wear a mask when working within a metre of the patient.
- Transport the patient out of the room only when necessary, and place a surgical mask on the patient if possible.

Contact precautions

- Use a private room, if available. Wear a mask when working within a metre of the patient.
- Transport the patient out of the room only when necessary, and place a surgical mask on the patient if possible.
- Wear a gown if contact with an infectious agent is likely or the patient has diarrhoea, an ileostomy, colostomy or wound drainage that is not contained by a dressing (Morton, Fontaine, Hudak & Gallo 2005: 1140).

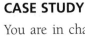

CASE STUDY

You are in charge of a health care institution. You receive daily reports from each department. The nurse in charge of the Emergency Department reports the admission of 20 patients, including a patient with these symptoms: itching; skin lesions; upper respiratory infection, with fever and shock. Blood cultures were taken for laboratory investigation, and family members confirm that the patient had eaten a dead animal.

Questions

1. Which disease(s) could you suspect?
2. Describe your instructions regarding standard precautions for treating this patient in the ward.
3. How could this disease spread?

Application to your own context

- Discuss infection control policies and their implementation with your infection control officer.
- Using the guidelines supplied in this chapter, draw up a policy for precautions for your unit or hospital.

TIPS FOR NURSES

Always familiarise yourself with the infection control measures in your health services, and consult with an infection control expert if you are not sure.

CONCLUSION

In South Africa the health system and population have changed substantially during the last decade. The practice of infection control has also evolved and all health care professionals must keep up to date with the latest knowledge and skills in infection control initiatives. Infections have increased during the last decade – new, more virulent infections now exist, in particular because of the increased access to medicine and the low literacy level of health care users. In response, infection control needs to be more flexible and innovative.

Infection control in hospitals and health services is all about the protection of the patients and the health professionals. As shown in Figure 1.1, it is important to think of the patient as the most important factor, surrounded by the factors that can affect them in the hospital environment.

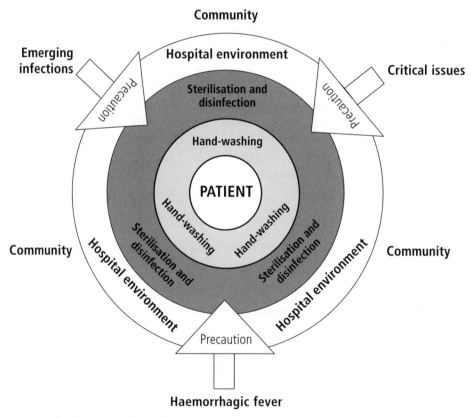

Figure 1.1 Infection control model

Referring to the figure, it is clear that you can protect the patient from nosocomial infections by:
- practising and promoting hand-washing before and after touching the patient (see Chapter Two)

- ensuring that all equipment is effectively sterilised, and that all sterilisation and disinfection procedures are of a high standard (see Chapter Three)
- being aware of the environmental aspects of a hospital that are vulnerable to the spread of infection, as well as conducting careful surveillance (see Chapter Four)
- ensuring that appropriate precaution procedures are in place and well known by all health professionals regarding critical issues such as urinary tract infections, surgical site infection, bloodstream infections and pneumonia (see Chapter Five)
- putting effective precautions in place regarding haemorrhagic fevers (see Chapter Six)
- emphasising the importance of infection control precautions regarding emerging diseases such as SARS, XDR TB, MDR TB and avian flu (see Chapter Seven).

SELF-ASSESSMENT

Before moving on to the next chapter, make sure that you can discuss the following key concepts and their application in your context with a colleague:
- Discuss standard precaution measures.
- Identify the contributing factors to infectious diseases in your particular health system and describe them using applicable examples.
- Consider how you would minimise the infection reservoirs in your hospital.

FURTHER READING AND WEB RESOURCES

Weaving, P. and Cooper, T. 2006. Infection control is everyone's business. *Nursing Management*, 12(10).

Ziady, L. E. and Small, N. 2004. *Prevent and control infection*. Cape Town: Juta.

CHAPTER TWO

Hand-washing in health care organisations

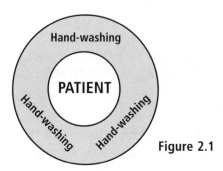

Figure 2.1

'What, will these hands ne'er be clean?'
Lady Macbeth, *Macbeth* (William Shakespeare)

Learning outcomes

Upon completion of this chapter, you should be able to:

- assess your hand hygiene practices and those of your colleagues
- give feedback to health care workers on their competencies regarding hand-washing in the health care setting
- identify the correct hand hygiene method for the various infections
- know how to do a surgical hand scrub in preparation for a surgical procedure.

Learning assumed to be in place

To gain the most benefit from this chapter, you should already have the following knowledge and skills:

- Knowledge on the different infective diseases in a health care setting.
- Knowledge of the history of infection control and related problems since Semmelweis's time.

Key ethical considerations

- Health professionals have to ensure that improved quality care is provided.
- The patient's rights must be upheld by each health professional.
- Patients have the right to a healthy and safe environment, free from the risk of nosocomial infections.

Key legislative considerations

- All health professionals are governed by Acts and regulations, such as the *National Health Act (61 of 2003)*.
- Nurses have a legal obligation to comply with the Acts regulating their practice as professional nurses, for example the *Nursing Act, 2005 (Act 33 of 2005)*.
- The *Occupational Health and Safety Act (85 of 1993, Section 8(1))* guides the employer to provide a safe environment for health professionals and to ensure that equipment and facilities help nurses and doctors to render safe patient care.
- *Disinfectant Act, 1972*, and relevant regulations. Health professionals are fully accountable for their acts and effective hand-washing practices need to be complied with in all circumstances when patients are cared for.

Important terms

- Alcohol-based hand-rub is a preparation containing alcohol that is designed for application to the hands. It is used for reducing the number of viable micro-organisms on the hands, and usually contains 60–95% ethanol or isopropanol.
- Anti-microbial agent is applied to the hands or skin to reduce the number of microbial flora. Examples of such agents are alcohols and chlorhexidine.
- Antiseptic hand-washing is the process of washing the hands with soap and water or other detergents containing an antiseptic agent such as alcohol, chlorhexidine, triclosan or other antiseptics.
- Antiseptic hand-rubbing entails applying an antiseptic hand-rub to all surfaces of the hands to reduce the number of micro-organisms.
- Decontamination of hands means reducing the bacterial counts on the hands.

> - A detergent is a compound that possesses a cleaning action; the term 'soap' is used to refer to such detergents.

- Hand antisepsis refers to an antiseptic hand-wash or antiseptic hand-rub.

- Hand hygiene is a general term that applies to hand-washing, antiseptic hand-washing, antiseptic hand-rub and a surgical hand antisepsis.

- Plain soap refers to a detergent that does not contain anti-microbial agents.

- Surgical hand antisepsis is an antiseptic hand-wash or antiseptic hand-rub performed pre-operatively by surgical personnel to eliminate transient flora.

- A waterless antiseptic agent is an antiseptic agent that does not require the use of exogenous water (Centre of Disease Control (CDC) 2002: 3).

- A moiety is each one of the parts into which something is or can be divided.

INTRODUCTION

In 1846, Ignaz Semmelweis observed that babies that were delivered by medical students and physicians in the first clinic at the general hospital of Vienna consistently had a higher mortality rate than those that were delivered by midwives in the second clinic. He believed that the puerperal fever that affected the mothers who gave birth to these babies was caused by 'cadaverous particles' transmitted from the autopsies to the obstetrics ward via the hands of the students and physicians. He insisted that they wash their hands between each patient contact, and as a result the mortality rate in the first clinic dropped dramatically. Semmelweis's intervention represents the first evidence that cleansing of hands between patient contacts may reduce the nosocomial infection rates in hospitals and health care organisations (CDC 2002: 1; Baron, Baron & Perrella 2006: 129–34).

Hand-washing and hand-washing techniques received attention throughout the 20th century and even today new developments and solutions for hand-washing continue to emerge. Research and systematic reviews have been done to inform us of effective hand hygiene standards for health care workers.

TRANSMISSION OF PATHOGENS

In order for you to understand hand-washing practices, we must revise the normal skin and its functions. The primary functions of our skin are to:
- reduce water loss
- provide protection against abrasive action and micro-organisms
- act as a permeability barrier to the environment.

Transient flora are the organisms most frequently associated with nosocomial infections. Resident flora, which are attached to the deeper layers of the skin, are more resistant to removal, and less likely to cause infections. Health care workers' hands may become persistently colonised with pathogenic flora as a result of contact with infected patients and substances.

During transmission of health care-associated pathogens from one patient to another via the hands of doctors, nurses, ancillary health care professionals, students and others, the following sequence of events takes place:

1. Organisms are present on the patient's skin and transferred to the health care worker's hands.
2. The organisms are capable of surviving for at least several minutes on the hands.
3. Hand-washing or hand antisepsis by the health professional is inadequate or omitted entirely, or the hand hygiene agent is inappropriate.
4. The health professional's contaminated hands come into direct contact with another patient, or into contact with an object that will come into direct contact with the patient (CDC 2002: 4).

Health care pathogens can be recovered not only from infected or draining wounds, but also from frequently colonised areas of normal intact patient skin. The perineal or inguinal areas are usually the most heavily colonised, though axillae, trunk and upper extremities, including the hands, are also frequently colonised with organisms such as *S. aureus*, *Proteus mirabilis*, *Klebsiella* spp. and *Acinetobacter* spp. Persons with diabetes, patients undergoing dialysis for chronic renal failure, and those with chronic dermatitis are all likely to have areas of intact skin colonised with *S. aureus*. During a cleaning activity hands could be contaminated, for example lifting a patient; taking a patient's pulse, blood pressure or oral temperature; or touching a patient's hand or shoulder. Health care workers' hands can also be contaminated during activities that involve direct patient contact, wound care, intravascular catheter care, respiratory tract care and handling the secretions of the patient. Examples of organisms that can contaminate the health care worker's hands during these activities are gram-negative bacilli, *S. aureus*, enterococci or *C. difficile* (CDC 2002: 4–5).

FACTORS INFLUENCING ADHERENCE TO HAND HYGIENE PRACTICES

Outbreak investigations have indicated an association between nosocomial infections, understaffing or overcrowding, where the association was consistently linked to poor adherence to hand hygiene. Thus, understaffing of nurses can facilitate the spread of MRSA in intensive care areas. In an outbreak of *Enterobacter cloacae* in a neonatal intensive care unit (ICU), the daily number of hospitalised children was above the maximum capacity of the unit, resulting in an available space per child that was below the current recommendations for safe and quality patient care. Furthermore, the number of staff members on duty was substantially less than the number required by the workload, which also resulted in relaxed attention paid to basic infection control measures. Adherence to hand hygiene practices dropped to 25% during peak workload times, but increased to 70% after the overcrowding period (CDC 2002: 6).

There are various reasons for health care workers failing to comply with hand hygiene practices. Generally, the reasons can be divided into three categories, namely:
1. Observed risk factors to poor adherence.
2. Self-reported factors of poor adherence.
3. Perceived barriers to adherence (CDC 2002: 23).

Observed risk factors for poor adherence

- The status of a health care worker, such as a physician rather than a nurse.
- Nursing auxiliary status, rather than that of a professional nurse.
- Males do not wash their hands as regularly as females do.
- Work performed in ICU.
- Work performed during the week.
- The wearing of gloves and gowns.
- Automated sinks.
- Activities with high risk of cross-infection.
- High number of opportunities for hand-washing per hour of patient care.

Self-reported factors of poor adherence

- Irritation and dryness of hands after use of the hand-washing agent.
- Inconveniently located sinks.
- Lack of soap and paper towels.
- Lack of time or opportunity.
- Understaffing and overcrowding of unit.
- Patients' needs.
- Low risk of cross-infection.
- The wearing of gloves and the belief that glove use obviates the need for hand-washing.
- Lack of knowledge.
- Forgetfulness.
- Lack of role modelling from other colleagues and health care team members.
- Scepticism towards hand-washing.
- Disagreement with hand-washing protocols.
- Lack of evidence-based knowledge available on hand-washing procedures.

Perceived barriers to adherence

- Lack of involvement of all staff members in hand hygiene promotion.
- Lack of role models.
- Lack of institutional priority.
- Lack of reward for compliers.
- Lack of safe climate in the institution.

HAND HYGIENE GUIDELINES

Hand-cleaning preparations are mainly available in plain soap, anti-microbial hand-washing soap and alcohol hand-rubs. The choice of the hand decontamination to be used must be based on the need to remove transient and resident flora from the hands.

Plain soap

In a study by Ehrenkranz and Alfonso (1991), as cited in the CDC (2002: 8), hand-washing with plain soap was seen to fail to remove pathogens from the hands of hospital staff, and the practice of washing hands with plain soap only was concluded to result in paradoxical increases in bacterial counts on the skin. Plain soap can also become contaminated with organisms and may result in colonising the hands of health care workers with gram-negative bacilli.

Alcohols

The majority of alcohol-based hand antiseptics contain isopropanol, ethanol, n-propanol or a combination of these. Alcohols have effective in vitro germicidal activity against gram-positive and -negative bacteria, including MRSA, mycobacterium TB and various fungi. Hepatitis B is an enveloped virus that is killed by 60–70% alcohol.

The efficiency of alcohol-based products is affected by certain factors:
• Contact time.
• Volume of alcohol used.
• Whether or not the hands are wet when alcohol is applied.

The application of small volumes, such as 0.5 ml, of alcohol to the hands is more effective than washing the hands with plain soap and water. It was found that 1 ml of alcohol was substantially less effective than 3 ml. The exact or ideal volume of alcohol to the hands is not known, but if the hands feel dry after being rubbed together for 15 seconds the amount of alcohol was insufficient. Frequent use of alcohol-based agents on the hands may cause dryness of skin, and emollients should be added to the alcohol skin-rub to prevent this, for example 1–3% glycerol (Picheansathian 2004: 6–7).

Chlorhexidine

The anti-microbial activity of chlorhexidine is likely attributable to attachment to and subsequent disruption of cytoplasmic membranes, resulting in precipitation of cellular contents (CDC 2002: 13). Chlorhexidine has effective activity against gram-positive bacteria, somewhat less effective activity against gram-negative bacteria and fungi, and minimally effective activity against TB. Chlorhexidine is not sporicidal. It has effective in vitro activity against enveloped viruses such as herpes simplex,

HIV, cytomegalovirus and influenza, with substantially less effective activity against rotavirus, adenovirus and enteroviruses.

Chloroxylenol

Chloroxylenol is a halogen-substituted phenolic compound that has been used as a preservative in cosmetics and other products. It has effective in vitro activity against gram-positive organisms, fairly effective activity against gram-negative bacteria, mycobacterium and viruses, and less effective activity against *Pseudomonas aeruginosa*.

Hexachlorophene

Hexachlorophene is a biphenol composed of two phenolic groups and three chlorine moieties (CDC 2002: 14). It is bacteriostatic, and has effective activity against *S. aureus* but relatively ineffective activity against gram-negative bacteria, fungi and mycobacterium.

Iodine and iodophors

Iodine has been recognised as an effective antiseptic since the 1800s, but it causes irritation and discolouration of the skin. Iodine and iodophors have bactericidal activity against gram-positive, gram-negative and certain spore-forming bacteria.

Quaternary ammonium compounds

These are primarily bacteriostatic and fungistatic. Although they are microbicidal, they are more active against gram-positive than against gram-negative bacteria.

Triclosan

Triclosan is a non-ionic, colourless substance that was developed in the 1960s. It has a broad range of anti-microbial activities, and is often bacteriostatic. However, it must be emphasised that Triclosan lacks potent activity against gram-negative bacilli.

Surgical hand antisepsis

Traditionally, surgical staff were required to scrub their hands for 10 minutes pre-operatively, which frequently led to skin damage. Scrubbing with a brush was also required, but this practice can also damage the skin and result in an increased shedding of bacteria from the hands. It is now clear that the two-stage surgical scrub is the practice of choice – use of antiseptic detergent is followed by application of an alcohol hand-rub. The initial one- to two-minute scrub with 4% chlorhexidine gluconate, or povidone-iodine, followed by an application of an alcohol-based product has proved to be more effective than a five-minute scrub with an antiseptic detergent alone (CDC 2002: 18).

HAND HYGIENE IN THE CASE OF SPECIFIC ORGANISMS

Staff's hands are the most common vehicle by which micro-organisms are transmitted between patients. Hands are frequently implicated as the route of transmission in outbreaks of infection in health care facilities. It is a generally accepted fact that staff's hands in clinical settings are frequently colonised with pathogens and that hand-washing is essential in removing micro-organisms from the hands in order to avoid cross-infection. The organisms, which in most cases cause serious outbreaks in hospitals settings, are *C. difficile* and MRSA.

Clostridium difficile and *Bacillus anthracis*

The widespread prevalence of health care-associated diarrhoea caused by *C. difficile* worldwide, and the *Bacillus anthracis* infections associated with contaminated items sent through the mail in the United States, has raised concerns regarding the activity of antiseptics against spore-forming bacteria. *C. difficile* is an aerobic gram-positive bacterium that was first identified and described in 1935. It has now become the most frequent agent for nosocomial-associated diarrhoea.

The clinical symptom is mainly diarrhoea, which usually starts 5 to 10 days after antibiotic therapy is commenced. It ranges from mild to severe, foul-smelling diarrhoea containing blood/mucus, fever, leucocytosis and abdominal pain. In the majority of cases, the illness is mild and full recovery is usual. Immunocompromised patients and the elderly may become seriously ill with dehydration. Occasionally, patients may develop a severe form of the disease, called 'pseudomembranous colitis'. Complications include pancolitis, toxic megacolon, perforation or endotoxin shock.

The treatment for *C. difficile* enterocolitis includes three basic strategies:
1. Discontinue or change the antibiotics that affected the patient's gut interflora, and replace with an antibiotic that is less associated with enterocolitis.
2. Avoid anti-peristaltic medication, which results in the retention of the pathogen and possibly a worsened enterocolitis-associated necrosis of the colon. Rehydration of the patient usually results in rapid improvement.
3. Initiate specific antibiotic therapy soon after diagnosis, and administer oral metronidazole at 400 mg 8 hourly for 10 days. If metronidazole is not effective, prescribe oral vancomycin 125 mg 6 hourly for 10 days (Damani 2006: 147).

Hands can become contaminated by direct contact with patients who are colonised or infected with *C. difficile*, or by contact with spores in a contaminated environment. Therefore, strict hand hygiene of health professionals before and after patient contact remains the most effective measure of preventing cross-infection. The patient's immediate environment and other areas where spores may accumulate – such as the sluice, commodes, toilets, bedpans, sinks and high-touch surfaces in the patient's bathroom – must be cleaned and disinfected frequently. Chlorine-containing chemicals should be used for such environmental cleaning (Damani 2006: 147–9).

However, none of the agents for hand decontamination described above facilitates the physical removal of *C. difficile* or *Bacillus anthracis* spores. Health care workers must be encouraged to wear gloves when handling patients with *C. difficile*-associated diarrhoea. After removal of the gloves, hands must be washed with soap and water and disinfected with an alcohol-based hand-rub.

Methicillin-resistant *Staphylococcus aureus* infection

Endemic MRSA adds to the burden of nosocomial sepsis, costs more per patient than methicillin-sensitive *S. aureus* infection, and predicts poorer patient outcomes (Johnson, Martin, Burrell, et al. 2005: 509). The most significant mode of transmission of MRSA within health organisations appears to be poor hand hygiene. Once introduced into a hospital, MRSA can spread quickly and colonise many staff members and patients. This alone suggests that health care workers must improve hand hygiene and equipment cleaning methods in their hospital. The introduction of alcohol/chlorhexidine hand-rubs, combined with education and motivational programmes, can improve hand hygiene compliance and reduce the number of nosocomial infections.

SIGNIFICANT ASPECTS OF HAND-WASHING COMPLIANCE

There are several aspects of importance in health professionals' hand-washing compliance. These professionals need to pay attention to the indications for hand-washing – the technique, skin health, standards for hand hygiene, gloving practices, and state of fingernails and jewellery.

Indications for hand hygiene

- Contact with a patient's intact skin – for example taking blood pressure, temperature and pulse, and conducting physical examination of a patient.
- Contact with environmental surfaces in the immediate vicinity of the patient.
- Following removal of gloves.

Techniques for hand hygiene

- Attention must be paid to the amount of hand hygiene solution.
- Duration of the hand hygiene procedure must be within the CDC guideline of one to two minutes.
- Selection of hand hygiene agents, alcohol-based hand-rubs, soap (antiseptic and detergents) must be done carefully. Figure 2.2 and Table 2.1 show the hand-washing technique.

Methods of hand skin maintenance

- Lotions and creams can prevent or minimise skin dryness and irritation caused by detergents.

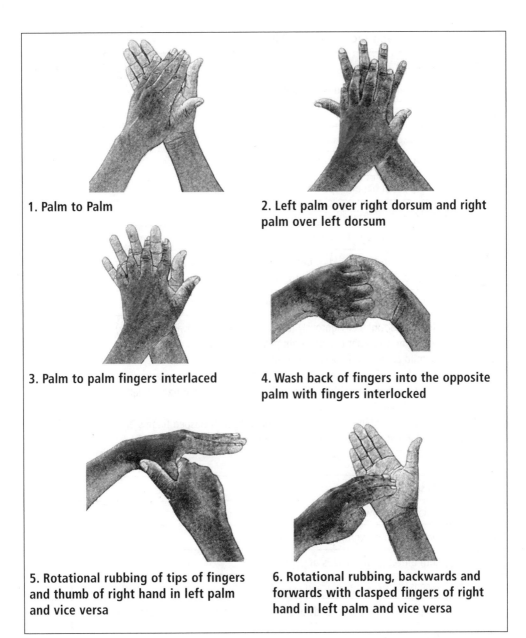

1. Palm to Palm

2. Left palm over right dorsum and right palm over left dorsum

3. Palm to palm fingers interlaced

4. Wash back of fingers into the opposite palm with fingers interlocked

5. Rotational rubbing of tips of fingers and thumb of right hand in left palm and vice versa

6. Rotational rubbing, backwards and forwards with clasped fingers of right hand in left palm and vice versa

Figure 2.2 Hand-washing technique

- Health professionals should use acceptable lotions or creams to protect the skin of their hands.
- A recommended schedule for applying lotions and creams should be in place.

Table 2.1 Hand-washing technique checklist

Number	Criteria	Score
1	Short nails; no cracked nail polish	
2	No rings or wristwatches	
3	Check soap for expiry date	
4	Check paper towel	
5	Check pedal bin and open it	
6	*Soap:* Contact with soap and with lather	
7	Use continuously running water	
8	*Position hands to avoid contamination of arms:* Hold hands down so that water drains from fingertips into sink	
9	Avoid splashing onto clothing and floor	
10 a b c d e	Rub hands together vigorously (as shown in Figure 2.1: Palm to palm) Left palm over right dorsum, right palm over left dorsum Palm to palm with fingers interlaced Wash back of fingers into the opposite palm with fingers interlocked Rotational rubbing of tips of fingers and thumb of right hand in left palm, then left hand in right palm Rotational rubbing, backwards and forwards with clasped fingers of right hand in left palm, then left hand in right palm (Pearce 1997: 119)	
11	Use friction on all surfaces	
12	Rinse hands thoroughly	
13	Hold hands down to rinse	
14	Dry hands thoroughly	
15	Turn off taps with elbows or paper towel	
16	Dispose of paper towel using pedal bin	
17	Keep hands away from body and above waist throughout the procedure	
18	Apply alcohol-based product on hands	

Expectations of care managers

- Written statements regarding the value of, and support for, hand hygiene adherence must be made available.
- Role models should demonstrate adherence to hand hygiene procedures.

Indications for, and limitations of, glove use

- Hand contamination may occur as a result of undetected holes in gloves.
- Contamination may occur during glove removal.
- Wearing gloves does not replace the need for hand-washing.
- Failure to remove gloves after caring for patients may lead to cross-infection.

The state of fingernails and jewellery

Freshly applied nail polish does not increase the number of bacteria, but chipped nail polish supports growth of larger numbers of organisms on the fingernails. Health care workers who wear artificial nails are more likely to harbour gram-negative pathogens on their fingertips than those who do not wear artificial nails. An outbreak of *P. aeruginosa* in a neonatal ICU was attributed to two nurses, one of whom had long natural nails and the other of whom had long artificial nails carrying the implicated strains of *Pseudomonas spp.* on their hands. Personnel wearing artificial nails have also been epidemiologically implicated in several other outbreaks of infection caused by gram-negative bacilli.

Furthermore, it is clear that the skin under rings is more heavily colonised than comparable areas of the skin on fingers without rings. Several studies indicated that nurses who wear rings were responsible for *S. aureus* infections and other gram-negative bacilli infections in the ICU (CDC 2002: 30).

CASE STUDY

Do you remember the 2005 case of the babies who died in Mahatma Gandhi Hospital in KwaZulu-Natal? The babies all died as a result of *Klebsiella spp.* infection. The case was reported only after seven babies died.

Questions

1. Write down a description of the case and a suggestion of the person(s) responsible for the babies' deaths.
2. What do you think the nurses could have done more effectively?

Application to your own context

What will you do to prevent such a thing from happening in your unit or your hospital? Remember, infection control is everyone's business!

TIPS FOR NURSES

- Wash your hands when they are visibly dirty or contaminated with bodily fluids.
- If hands are not visibly soiled, use an alcohol-based hand-rub for routine decontamination of hands.

- Decontaminate hands before and after direct patient contact.
- Decontaminate hands after removing gloves.
- When using an alcohol-rub, apply the product to the palm of one hand and rub your hands together, covering all surfaces of hands and fingers, until your hands are dry.
- When washing hands with soap and water, wet them first with water, apply soap and rub hands together vigorously for at least 15 seconds, covering all surfaces of the hands and fingers. Rinse your hands with water and dry them thoroughly with a disposable towel.
- Remove rings, watch and bracelets before beginning a surgical hand scrub.
- Remove debris from under the fingernails using a nail cleaner under running water.
- Surgical hand antisepsis using an anti-microbial soap or an alcohol-based hand-rub with persistent activity is recommended before sterile gloves are put on (Ziady & Small 2004: 178).

PRECAUTIONS

Keep the following in mind:
- Always be familiar with the infection control measures in your health services.
- Make sure you know the current infection control and hand hygiene method used in your health care institution.
- Always adhere to the set standards for infection control.
- Be a role model for other nurses and health care workers regarding hand hygiene.
- Provide accessible alcohol-based hand-rub for all health care workers.
- Ask if you are not sure.

CONCLUSION

Health care organisations must test the performance indicators from time to time to establish how they are doing regarding infection control practices. It is important to periodically monitor, and record adherence to, the number of hand hygiene episodes performed by personnel in the hospitals by ward and services, and give feedback to staff on their performance. Moreover, the amount of alcohol-based hand-rub used by health care workers must be monitored per patient per day. Adherence to infection control policies regarding nails, artificial nails and jewellery must also be monitored. When outbreaks of infection occur, assessment of the adequacy of all health care workers' hand hygiene practices must be done.

SELF-ASSESSMENT

Before moving on to the next chapter, make sure that you can discuss the following key concepts and their application in your context with a colleague:

- Ask your colleague to assess your hand hygiene for one day. Listen to their feedback and, if necessary, improve your hand hygiene practice.
- Look at your hands closely in the light of all the factors we have discussed in this chapter. Assess the risk you may pose to patients with your hands and your hand hygiene practices.
- You are one of the nurses allocated to do the wound round today. You consult the protocol file and find that there is no protocol for a hand-washing technique. Draw up such a protocol, ensuring that it complies with the CDC infection control guidelines.

FURTHER READING AND WEB RESOURCES

http://www.cdc.gov/ncidod/hip
http://www.med.upenn.edu
http://www.hopisafe.ch

CHAPTER THREE

Disinfection and sterilisation

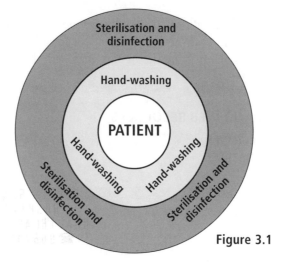

Figure 3.1

Learning outcomes

Upon completion of this chapter, you should be able to:

- identify methods of decontamination
- explain environmental cleaning in a hospital
- describe the procedure for terminal cleaning of a hospital room once an infective patient has been discharged
- identify the procedure for the management of blood spills in a hospital
- describe the procedure for decontamination of suction equipment in a hospital
- explain the different disinfection procedures for individual items and equipment following patient use in a hospital.

Learning assumed to be in place

To gain the most benefit from this chapter, you should already have the following knowledge and skills:

- Basic infection control knowledge with regard to a hospital.
- Basic knowledge of cleaning and disinfection in a hospital.

Key ethical considerations

- There should be adequate clean water and effective waste disposal and sanitation services.
- The principle of 'Do no harm' to the patient not only applies throughout this book, it is also essential during the re-use of equipment for patient care and when the environment is cleaned, so that patients are protected against nosocomial infections.

Key legislative considerations

- All health care workers are governed by Acts and regulations, such as the *National Health Act (61 of 2003)*.
- Nurses have a legal obligation to comply with the Acts regulating their practice as professional nurses, for example the *Nursing Act (33 of 2005)*, and they are expected to fulfil their professional and contractual obligations diligently and respectfully regarding the safety of patients.
- The *Occupational Health and Safety Act (85 of 1993, Section 8(1))*.

Important terms

- Decontamination is categorised into three levels, namely, sterilisation, disinfection and cleaning. It is furthermore divided into three categories of risk, namely:
  - high – such as surgical instruments, which need sterilisation
  - medium – for example endoscopes, bedpans and crockery, which need sterilisation
  - low – such as wash bowls and mattresses, which simply need normal cleaning.
- Sterilisation is the process of completely destroying or removing all micro-organisms, including bacterial spores.
- Disinfection is the process that reduces the number of micro-organisms to a level at which they are not harmful, but at which spores are not usually destroyed.

>

> • Cleaning of instruments before decontamination is an essential procedure. It allows for the physical removal of micro-organisms, which prevents inactivation of the disinfectant by organic matter and allows complete surface contact during further decontamination procedures.
>
> • Antiseptics are chemicals used to kill microbes on body surfaces.
>
> • Aseptic means free of organisms.
>
> • Terminal cleaning should be performed of a hospital room in which the discharged patient was isolated for an infection.

INTRODUCTION

The transmission of infection in association with equipment has been a problem in health care facilities ever since micro-organisms were identified as a possible source of infection. Inadequate decontamination has frequently been responsible for infection outbreaks in these facilities. Safe decontamination of equipment between patient uses is the cornerstone of good infection control practices. The environment is commonly perceived as a more significant source of infection than evidence proves. Microbes cannot multiply in dry environments – most die rapidly on surfaces or in air. Where moisture is present, for example in food, solutions or equipment containing water, the microbiological hazard is greater.

The procedure for terminal cleaning following patient discharge, the management of blood spills and infectious spills, and the disinfection of certain items used in hospitals will all be discussed in this chapter from the viewpoint of the sister-in-charge of a unit.

PROCEDURE FOR TERMINAL CLEANING

According to Damani (2006: 75), fumigation of the room is not necessary. Domestic staff should wear appropriate personal protective equipment, such as household gloves and disposable plastic aprons. All disposable items must be discarded. Clinical waste must be sealed in waste bags before being taken out of the room and should be disposed of according to local policies. Items from the central sterilisation supply department (CSSD) should be cleaned and then sent to the CSSD for sterilisation. Linen must be placed in appropriate linen bags and sealed before being taken away from the area. Dusting of high ledges, windows, curtain rails, fixtures, fittings, taps, sinks and door handles must be done using wet dusting. The floor must be vacuum-cleaned with a high filter mechanism and washed with detergent, rinsed and left to dry thoroughly. The bed should be wiped with warm water and a detergent such as hypochlorite 1:1 000, and left to dry thoroughly. Windows can be opened if required. The next patient should be admitted only when all surfaces are dry.

MANAGEMENT OF BLOOD SPILLS AND INFECTIOUS SPILLS

There is no documented evidence showing that any blood-borne virus – HIV, or hepatitis B or C – has been transmitted from an environmental surface. Nonetheless, prompt removal of a spill and surface disinfection of an area contaminated by either blood or bodily fluids are needed as part of effective infection control practices.

The procedure for cleaning splashes and spills is as follows:
• Wear non-sterile gloves.
• Wipe the area immediately with paper towel soaked in hypochlorite.
• Rinse the area with water.
• Dry the surface.
• Discard the gloves and paper towel as clinical waste.
• Wash and dry your hands immediately.

The procedure for cleaning large spills is as follows:
• Wear non-sterile gloves.
• Sprinkle the spill with approved disinfectant or NaDCC granules until the fluid is absorbed. For very large spills, cover the spillage with paper towels to absorb all liquid and carefully pour hypochlorite solution on the area.
• Leave the spill area for a contact period of about three minutes, to allow disinfection.
• Scoop up the absorbed granules or paper towels and discard in the prescribed waste bag (yellow) as clinical waste.
• Wipe the surface with fresh hypochlorite and rinse with clean water.
• Dry the surface.
• Remove the gloves and discard them and the paper towel as clinical waste.
• Wash and dry your hands immediately (Damani 2006: 76).

DISINFECTION OF ITEMS USED IN HOSPITAL

Equipment and items that have been contaminated by contact or other means must be decontaminated prior to use on the next patient.

Procedural guidelines for cleaning and disinfecting suction equipment:
• Suction unit can either be fixed and re-useable, or portable and usually used with re-useable suction jar.
• Suction tubing and catheters are disposable.
• Suction containers or reservoirs can be disposable or non-disposable.
• When emptying the non-disposable suction jar the following principles apply:
  – Wear plastic apron and household gloves.
  – Wear eye protection when patient is infectious or high-risk.
  – Wear high filtration mask if patient is diagnosed with TB.

- Disconnect jar from vacuum system.
- Carry jar carefully to sluice and pour gently into sluice.
- Flush away contents.
- Rinse jar, then wash with neutral pH detergent and hot water.
- Rinse again.
- Dry.
- Use weak solution of sodium bicarbonate to help remove mucus.
- Empty jar when full, and wash daily.
- Attach fresh tubing just prior to use.
- Routine use for disinfectant is needed for cleaning suction bottles, most importantly when the patient is infectious.
- If patient has TB, decontaminate jar.
- Use fresh single-use disposable suction catheter each time patient is suctioned (Damani 2006: 80).

Table 3.1 provides guidelines for decontamination of other items or sites. This is not a comprehensive list, it simply includes the most common items used in hospital units or clinics.

CASE STUDY

You are the sister-in-charge of a ward. You discover that the suction equipment is not decontaminated properly. You ask the nursing staff why this had not been done and they complain about the lack of a procedure regarding the cleaning of suction equipment.

Question

What is the most important point to remember when decontaminating equipment in a hospital or clinic?

Application to your own context

- Evaluate the decontamination procedure in your unit or clinic by using Table 3.1.
- Do you think nurses know enough about decontamination to be safe practitioners in hospital wards and clinics?

Table 3.1 Decontamination guidelines

Equipment or site	Method of decontamination
Airways and endotracheal tubes	Single use and disposable
Ampoules	Wipe neck with 70% isopropyl alcohol swab and allow to dry before opening or piercing
Arm splint	Wash with detergent, rinse and allow to dry
Baby's feeding bottles and teats	Use pre-sterilisation or heat-treated feeds. Non-disposable bottles must be washed thoroughly, rinsed and placed in fresh hypochlorite for at least 30 minutes. Chemical disinfectant should be used only when other methods are not available. Bottles should not be disinfected at ward level
Baths	Non-infected patients: Clean with detergent or use a non-abrasive cream cleanser to remove stain or scum, if needed. Rinse and dry Infected patients: Clean with chlorine-based agent or non-abrasive chlorine-releasing powder, rinse and dry
Beds and cots	Wash with detergent, rinse and dry. In the case of infected patients, use hypochlorite solution. Do not use phenolic disinfections on infant cots or incubators as residual fumes may cause respiratory irritation
Bedpans and urinals	Dispose after single use. If re-usable, heat-disinfect in a washer at 80 °C and store dry. Use gloves and plastic aprons when handling contaminated items from infected patients, or use disposable items
Bowls (washing)	Individual washbowls should be available for each patient. After use, wash the bowl with detergent, rinse and dry. In the case of an infected patient, clean and disinfect the bowl by wiping it with a disinfectant solution
Bowls (vomit)	Empty and rinse. Wash with detergent and hot water, rinse and dry. In the case of an infected patient, treat the bowls as washing bowls
Cardiac monitors, defibrillators and ECG equipment	If surface was in contact with patient, clean and disinfect it
Carpets	Suction-clean daily with a vacuum cleaner with an effective filter. Shampoo periodically
Cleaning equipment	Mops with detachable heads must be machine washed, thermally disinfected and dried daily. The mop bucket must be washed with detergent, rinsed and dried. The scrubbing machine must be drained after used and stored dry

>

Equipment or site	Method of decontamination
Commodes	Wash with detergent between use, and disinfect
Crockery and cutlery	Machine-wash with rinse temperature above 80 °C and dry, or hand-wash in detergent and hot water at 60 °C, rinse and dry
Drains	Clean regularly according to the policy of the hospital
Drip stands	Clean after each use
Duvets	Launder after each patient use
Endoscopes	Wash thoroughly, rinse and send dry to the CSSD for sterilisation. If used on a patient with tuberculosis, soak in 2% alkaline glutaraldehyde for over an hour
Enteral feeding lines	Single use and disposable
Floors (dry cleaning)	Vacuum-clean or use a dust-attracting mop. Never use brooms in patient areas
Floors (wet cleaning)	Wash with detergent solution. Disinfection is not required, but if contamination has occurred, disinfect and clean
Fixtures and fittings	In clinical areas, damp-dust daily with detergent
Haemodialysis machines	Clean and disinfect, paying attention to microbial quality of water and fluid pathway. Regular microbiological monitoring is essential
Humidifiers	Clean and sterilise between patients and fill with sterile water, which must be changed at least every 24 hours
Infant incubators	After use, wash all removable parts and clean with detergent. Clean and dry regularly
Instruments	Return to the CSSD for machine washing and sterilising
Razors and scissors	Surface disinfect with a 70% alcohol-impregnated wipe
Stethoscope	Surface disinfect after each use
Suction equipment	After each use the reservoir must be emptied in a sluice, washed with hot water and detergent, rinsed and stored dry (see also the longer 'Procedural guidelines for cleaning and disinfecting suction equipment', above)
Thermometers	Where possible single use, or patient-specific use. After use, wipe with 70% isopropyl alcohol-impregnated wipe and store dry
Trolleys (dressing, patient)	Clean and surface disinfect. If contaminated, clean and then use an alcohol-impregnated wipe

Equipment or site	Method of decontamination
Ventilators	Treat according to infection control policies of the hospital. Send for cleaning at the CSSD
X-ray equipment	Damp-dust with detergent solution, and if contaminated clean with alcohol-impregnated wipe

Source: Damani (2006: 81–9)

TIPS FOR NURSES

When you are unsure of a procedure, always consult with the infection control officer in your area or hospital. Remember the ethical code of 'Do no harm' to the patient when you need to decontaminate items for patient use. Pay attention to the following:

- Cleaning of instruments before decontamination is an essential part of infection control.
- Cleaning should always be carried out by trained staff.
- Machine-washing is the preferred option.
- Disinfection by either heat or chemicals will destroy micro-organisms but not bacterial spores.
- Remember that sterilisation is a process that achieves complete destruction of all micro-organisms, including bacterial spores.
- Remember that the outcome of a disinfection procedure is affected by the presence of organic material.
- Bear in mind the important aspects of concentration and contact time of decontamination agents, which determine the effectiveness of disinfection.

PRECAUTIONS

Always familiarise yourself with the infection risk from equipment in the health care setting. Be exceptionally careful when the risks are high for the patient to contract a nosocomial infection. The categories of risks are as follows:

- Critical or high-risk items come into close contact with a break in the skin or mucous membranes, or are introduced into a sterile body area. Single-use items are the safest in these cases.
- Semi-critical or intermediate risk items come into close contact with mucous membranes or bodily fluids. In certain cases, these items may be transferred to the high-risk category. Single-use items are the preferred option, but disinfection by heat is allowed.
- Non-critical or low-risk items are exposed to normal and intact skin. Cleaning and drying of these items is essential.
- Minimal-risk items are not exposed to the patient or their immediate environment. These items are unlikely to be contaminated with micro-organisms, for example lockers, walls, floors and ceilings.

CONCLUSION

Equipment and items that have been contaminated by contact with blood and high-risk bodily fluids or pathological specimens, or that have been exposed to patients in isolation, will require decontamination prior to being sent to the CSSD and other cleaning and disinfection departments. The sister-in-charge is responsible for ensuring that the correct procedures are followed, that policy implementation is done correctly and that the environment is safe for patients.

SELF-ASSESSMENT

Before moving on to the next chapter, make sure that you can discuss the following key concepts and their application in your context with a colleague:
- Decontamination.
- Sterilisation.
- Disinfection.
- Cleaning.
- Aseptic.
- Terminal cleaning.

FURTHER READING AND WEB RESOURCES

http://www.who.int/
http://www.cdc.gov/ncidod/hip
http://www.med.upenn.edu
http://www.hopisafe.ch
http://www.mosby.com/ajic
http://www.cdc.gov/ncidod/EID/index.htm
http://www.slackinc.com/general/iche
http://www.his.org.uk
http://www.icna.co.uk

CHAPTER FOUR

Environmental aspects of the prevention of nosocomial infection

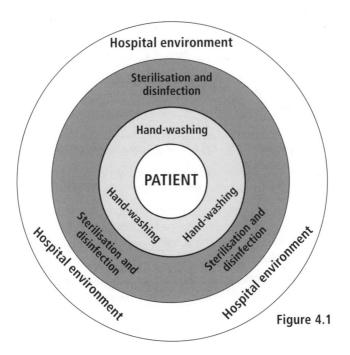

Figure 4.1

Learning outcomes

Upon completion of this chapter, you should be able to:

- know of aspects in the environment of a hospital that could lead to nosocomial infections
- know how to do surveillance in the hospital and your unit.

Learning assumed to be in place

To gain the most benefit from this chapter, you should already have the following knowledge and skills:

- Knowledge of nosocomial infections.
- Knowledge of the various precaution strategies for the different types of infections that can occur in a hospital.
- An understanding of the source of infection control.

Key ethical considerations

- Health care professionals are obliged to ensure that health care facilities are designed to allow easy and simple routine cleaning and disinfection.
- Health care professionals must prevent dust from collecting in all areas and in this regard the use of cupboards rather than shelves is recommended.
- Health care professionals must prevent infections from spreading in the hospital by implementing the guidelines on the handling of used, soiled and contaminated linen; waste management in the wards and pest control, and must report any infections to infection control officers.
- Health professionals must perform daily surveillance in order to identify and curb any nosocomial infection in order to prevent outbreak of disease in the hospital.

Key legislative considerations

- All health professionals are accountable for their actions and omissions during patient care in a hospital or health service. Accountability also implies that there is a conditional liability for actions. To accept accountability, you need to observe and examine a situation, as well as the various options available on which to base a decision.

> **Important terms**
>
> - Surveillance means different things to different people. In the context of this book, the term means collection, collation, analysis and dissemination of information related to health and health care organisations. The aim of surveillance is early identification of outbreaks or potential outbreaks in the hospital or community. Surveillance is conducted at various levels internationally, nationally and locally in each hospital or health care institution.

INTRODUCTION

Although the environment plays a limited role in the spread of nosocomial infections, a dirty patient area can promote cross-infection. The purpose of cleaning is to physically remove the dirt and micro-organisms from surfaces in order to prevent contamination from health worker to patient, and from patient to patient. In extremely vulnerable patient areas, such as infant and neonatal care units, and immunocompromised patient units, the environment does play a role in nosocomial infection spread, and therefore meticulous attention should be given to the cleanliness of these environments (Ziady & Small 2004: 140).

The current budget constraints and the outsourcing of cleaning services result in an overall deterioration in hospital hygiene in South Africa and elsewhere. In addition to reducing potential reservoirs for micro-organisms, environmental cleaning has a significant aesthetic purpose in hospitals and is crucial for enhancing patient confidence in the treatment they receive. Important environmental aspects are air, water, carpets, specialised patient care units, linen, flower arrangements and waste disposal (Damani 2006: 17–24). An efficient surveillance system, through which operative measures are implemented for identifying and managing the risk of outbreaks, is a crucial factor in an effective infection control programme in a health care organisation.

As we discussed in Chapter Two, meticulous hand-washing is essential in the prevention of transmission of micro-organisms from the environment to the patient. The use of alcohol-based, water-free hand antiseptics is suited for all health care organisations, in particular where hand-washing facilities are not readily available and water is scarce. All cleaning procedures should be defined and applied consistently throughout the hospital system. Cleaning personnel must be properly trained and supervised. Products for cleaning and decontamination should be used according to the health care facility's policies and procedures. Moreover, all products and procedures must be scientifically based. Environmental surfaces should be cleaned with a detergent when visibly soiled, and made aesthetically acceptable for patients and staff. The use of non-critical equipment should be dedicated to infected patients, and, if this is not possible, shared non-critical items must be cleaned and disinfected between patient use.

THE HOSPITAL ENVIRONMENT AND SPECIFIC INTERVENTIONS

The functional design of a health care facility should facilitate simple cleaning and disinfection procedures. Surfaces must be smooth and easy to clean, and at the same time surfaces must be protected from damage and made of impervious material. The environment poses a significant microbiological hazard where moisture is present, for example in food, solutions and water sources.

Air and water

The role of air in the spread of nosocomial infections must be examined from the perspective of organisms. For example, it is known that droplets of M.TB and varicella zoster, measles and influenza are transmitted through the air, and guidelines to reduce the risk of their spread must be implemented. Legionella pneumophila outbreaks have been associated with cooling systems and thus the systems must be properly maintained and cleaned frequently. However, efficient air management is not always possible in a health care organisation. If the organisation has air conditioners then the filters must be replaced frequently. Rooms with good airflow, such as those with open windows in rural hospitals, can also benefit from the use of extractor fans in cases of TB-infected patients, in order to lower the risk of TB transmission.

Contaminated water is a well-known source of nosocomial infection in health care organisations. Medical devices that use water – for example respirators and fibre-optic endoscopes – can be a source of infection and should be treated accordingly. Haemodialysis water has been clearly identified as a source of pyrogenic reactions and bacteraemia in kidney patients. Several types of bacteria are capable of surviving and multiplying in distilled and other water sources, all of which are used for haemodialysis. Water in undersourced areas can be made safer by solar disinfection through the use of solar box cookers that reach pasteurisation temperatures and boil the water for 10 minutes, and the equipment can be chemically disinfected.

Environmental surfaces

Walls and ceilings are not likely sources of contamination and infection of patients. These surfaces do not need disinfection, but should be cleaned periodically. Floors should be cleaned without the use of a disinfectant. No bodily fluids should be visible on any surface in a hospital. There is no definite evidence showing that carpets cause infection in a hospital. Nevertheless, hospital carpets should be washable, with waterproof backing and sealed joints. To prevent fungal growth, carpets must be dried properly. They should also not be laid in areas where bodily fluid spillage is likely to occur, such as in surgical and obstetric wards.

Linen

Bedlinen can become rapidly contaminated with skin scales and therefore frequent changing of linen is of limited value. Linen should be changed if it is soiled, wrinkled or contaminated with infected material. There are three categories of linen:

1. Used linen has come into contact with the patient.
2. Soiled linen is visibly dirty and stained with bodily fluids.
3. Contaminated linen has come into contact with infected patients.

Linen should never be sorted and shaken out in the patient area, and never be carried from one place to another. The used linen container should always be at hand. The filled linen containers should be sealed and stored away from clean linen and patients. Soiled linen must be separated from other linen and bagged according to the regulation of the health service, in colour-coded plastic bags. Linen used for patients with haemorrhagic fever should be double-bagged and incinerated, or autoclaved and discarded.

Linen should never be sorted and sluiced on the ward – this should be done in the laundry, according to the health service's regulations. Soiled linen should be machine-washed in the cold cycle before it is washed again, at a temperature of 90 °C. Curtains should be washed when visibly soiled or every six months, separately from bedlinen (Damani 2006: 17–24; Ziady & Small 2004: 150–2).

Plants and/or flowers

Hand-washing following the handling of flowers and potted plants will eliminate the risk of hand contamination in a hospital, although there is little evidence linking flowers to the spread of nosocomial infections.

Waste management

Most hospitals and health care institutions produce medical waste at a high rate. Plastic disposables are difficult to degrade or incinerate. In the light of the fact that preserving our environment and natural resources is a worldwide priority, the question that health care organisations must now ask is how to avoid producing waste rather than how to dispose of it. Currently, there is little evidence that medical waste constitutes a significant public hazard, but it is important that the legislation on waste disposal is complied with nonetheless. Medical waste must be contained to prevent leakage, and sharps must be discarded in puncture-resistant containers. Incineration, autoclaving, mechanical or chemical disinfection, microwave decontamination and compacting are all strategies for waste disposal that are available to health care organisations (Damani 2006: 304–8).

Pest control

A pest control strategy must in place in areas such as kitchens, cafeterias, laundries, sterile supply areas and operating rooms, as they are prone to infestation and can facilitate insect vector-borne infections. Pests require food, warmth, moisture, refuge and a means of entry. Therefore, hospital staff should keep food covered and get rid of spillage and waste immediately. Modern approaches to pest control management usually focus on:

- covering food sources
- excluding pests from the indoor environment
- applying pesticides as needed (Damani 2006: 312–13).

SURVEILLANCE SYSTEM

In the context of this book, surveillance implies the collection, collation, analysis and dissemination of information related to health and health care organisations. The aim of surveillance is early identification of outbreaks or potential outbreaks in the hospital or community. Surveillance is conducted at various levels internationally, nationally and locally.

The incidence rate of MRSA, *C. difficile*-associated diarrhoea (CDAD) and vancomycin-resistant enterococcus (VRE) is on the rise globally. Patients infected with anti-microbial-resistant bacteria have significant morbidity and mortality, with increased costs to health care facilities and taxpayers. Infection surveillance and control activities have been shown to be effective in reducing resistant pathogen rates in hospitals.

Important surveillance activities for health services should include the following:

- Infection statistics must be collected by ward, units or services.
- Infection statistics should be collected for particular anatomical sites and medical devices.
- Surgical site infection rates must be calculated and reported to surgeons.
- Surgical site infection rates must be calculated for clean procedures.
- Hospitalised patients must all be examined, and their charts should be reviewed for new infections.
- Infection control staff should contact physicians or nurses for reports of new infections.
- Infection control reports should be filled out by ward staff and sent to the infection control unit.
- Discharged patients and their doctors should be contacted in the case of a suspected infection.
- The charts of discharged patients should be reviewed by infection control staff.
- Statistical computer programs should be used to monitor and research infections (Zoutman & Ford 2005: 2).

PRINCIPLES OF INFECTION CONTROL

The principles are as follows:

- There should be a programme for teaching nursing and ancillary staff the current infection control practices. The infection control team should serve as the specialist's advisors by taking the leading role in the effective functioning of the infection control programme.
- Attendance records should be kept of all staff training on infection control practices.
- The effectiveness of infection control training should be monitored.
- Infection rates should be communicated to staff.
- Infection control officers should have direct authority to close a ward or a unit to further admissions.
- A precaution methods policy should be in place.
- An antibiotics policy should be in place.
- A comprehensive guide on prevention of infections should be in place (Zoutman & Ford 2005: 2).

INFECTION CONTROL ASSESSMENT GUIDE

Each institution should draw up a tool for ward/unit infection control evaluation. The evaluation could assist in providing a safe environment for staff and patients, and thus in preventing nosocomial infections from spreading. Aspects that should be included in such an evaluation are as follows:

1. Staff:
   a. Hygiene level.
   b. In-service education on infection control.
2. Patients:
   a. Number of patients with infections.
   b. List of patients with infections.
3. Patient environment/units/ward.
4. Equipment.
5. Isolation.
6. Bathrooms.
7. Toilets.
8. Doctor's rooms.
9. Injection room.
10. Duty room.
11. Nurses' station.
12. Emergency trolley.
13. Dressing room.
14. Passages.
15. Kit room.
16. Storerooms.

17. Chute area.
18. Sluice room.
19. Stockroom.
20. Cleaners' room.
21. Linen room.
22. Offices.
23. Kitchen area.
24. Tearoom.

MANAGEMENT OF AN OUTBREAK

An outbreak can be defined as the occurrence of disease at a rate greater than expected within a specific geographical area and over a defined period of time (Damani 2006: 30). Day-to-day surveillance is important in identifying nosocomial infections in a health service. Major outbreaks in hospitals, other services and communities require appropriate planning and management:

1. All health care facilities should have effective outbreak control plans.
2. Communication forms the cornerstone of successful handling of an outbreak.
3. Rapid recognition of an outbreak is one of the most significant objectives of outbreak control.
4. Investigation of the outbreak entails four basic steps:
   a. Description of the outbreak.
   b. Collection of data on the incident.
   c. Development of a hypothesis.
   d. Testing of the hypothesis with analytic epidemiology.
5. Speedy outbreak control and the introduction of preliminary control measures should be based on sound infection control principles, such as precaution-taking and effective hand-washing. Subsequent control plans should be based on the infection itself and on the number of cases.
6. Senior managers and all involved parties should communicate effectively about the outbreak.
7. Following the outbreak, the control committee should prepare a report, including aspects such as experiences of the participants, the shortfalls and difficulties, and revision of the outbreak control plan and any recommendations for improvement.

In order to investigate an outbreak, the relevant staff need to:
- conduct a background information study to establish the infection rate
- confirm the existence of the outbreak
- confirm the diagnosis of the outbreak, using the laboratory results
- create a case definition based on clinical evidence and laboratory results
- develop line listings by identifying and counting the cases or exposures to the infection

- constructing an epidemic curve, including the source of the outbreak – a bar diagram can aid clarity in this regard
- develop and test a hypothesis for the outbreak
- take immediate control measures, determining who is at risk and looking at changes that might affect the rate of infection, such as new staff, new procedures, laboratory results and staffing ratios in the hospital
- communicate information to hospital management and staff
- screen the hospital staff and environment
- write a comprehensive report, with an executive summary addressed to the relevant authorities
- implement long-term infection control procedures, once the particular outbreak is over, in order to prevent further outbreaks (Damani 2006: 33).

CASE STUDY

Infection control is emerging as a highly important aspect in health services today. Babies are dying because of lack of infection surveillance in hospitals. It seems as if the rural hospitals are more affected by nosocomial infections, where the patients died as a result of a hospital infection. A hospital was in the news in 2006 because seven newborn babies died of a Klebsiella infection. There was no infection control practice in this hospital and the hospital board decided to appoint an infection control nurse.

You are a newly qualified professional nurse and you are appointed at Mahatma Gandhi Hospital in KwaZulu-Natal as the infection control nurse. The hospital management commissioned you with the task of conducting surveillance in the hospital and you need to have an evaluation tool to assist you in this task.

Question

Draw up a comprehensive infection control evaluation instrument – that is, a checklist – for a neonatal ward regarding staffing issues and the hand-wash basins. Use the list above as a guide.

Application to your own context

- Consult with the infection control officers to ensure that your evaluation tool is relevant and up to date.
- Why do you think surveillance is important? Give reasons for your answer.
- What is the best method for handling the soiled linen of an infected patient? Describe the method and give reasons for your answer.

TIPS FOR NURSES

Be proactive and knowledgeable about infection control practices. Read widely on new infectious diseases and their management. Consult if you are not sure. Ensure that all staff members have access to the infection control policy and guidelines. Encourage every staff member to attend infection control workshops and training.

PRECAUTIONS

Infection control is an integral part of high quality health services. Identifying and managing the risks related to infection, monitoring the outcome and ensuring that appropriate procedures are in place are all functions that each health professional must perform. The risks of infection should be analysed, which includes identifying and quantifying infection hazards and the conditions under which infection occurs. Risk management entails the action implemented to eliminate the risks. Staff need to be informed of risks, which should further be monitored by assessment of the effectiveness of infection control measures that are in place in the health care facility.

CONCLUSION

Hospitals that have infection control practices in place are better able to combat nosocomial infections. It is essential that all staff members know the infection control practices and can report and consult in case of emergency. The better a hospital is prepared, the lower the risk of nosocomial infections.

SELF-ASSESSMENT

Before moving on to the next chapter, make sure that you can discuss the following key concepts and their application in your context with a colleague:
- Describe how you should handle sharps in your unit.
- Discuss the consequences of ignorance with regard to infection control.
- Discuss the factors contributing to infections in the hospital environment.

FURTHER READING AND WEB RESOURCES

Ziady, L. E. and Small, N. 2004. *Prevent and control infection.* Cape Town: Juta.

CHAPTER FIVE

Critical issues in infection control

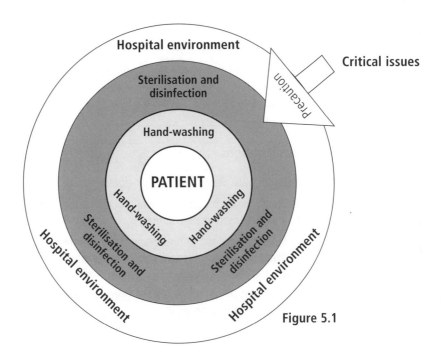

Figure 5.1

Learning outcomes

Upon completion of this chapter, you should be able to:

- assess your infection control practices with regard to surgical wounds, urinary tract catheters and intravenous (IV) catheters

- educate health care professionals on the principles of infection control for urinary tract catheters, surgical wounds and IV catheters

- demonstrate the correct procedure for insertion of a catheter into the urethra

- demonstrate the correct procedures for insertion of an IV catheter

- demonstrate the various wound types and the risks for infection in wounds

- assess your hospital's methods of decreasing ventilator-associated pneumonia (VAP).

Learning assumed to be in place

To gain the most benefit from this chapter, you should already have the following knowledge and skills:

- Knowledge of basic effective hygiene.
- Knowledge of aseptic procedures.
- Knowledge of infectious disease prevention in a hospital.
- Knowledge of sterilisation and disinfection methods.

Key ethical considerations

- Health professionals must wash their hands before inserting an IV catheter.
- Health professionals must prevent bacteria from entering the bladder of the catheterised patient at the time of insertion.
- Health professionals are obliged to prevent any harm or infection to patients who are on mechanically assisted ventilation, such as those who are intubated or have endotracheal and tracheotomy tubes.
- All health professionals should know the key elements for minimising the risk of surgical wound infections in a hospital.

Key legislative considerations

Health professionals are accountable for their actions and omissions and therefore must utilise all their skills and knowledge to prevent infections, such as bloodstream, urinary tract, respiratory and surgical wound infection.

Important terms

- Urinary tract infections are the most common infection acquired in a hospital or health service.
- Surgical site infections are superficial and stem from bacterial inoculation during surgery. They are caused by gram-positive cocci, including *S. aureus*, *Staphylococcus epidermidis* and enterococcus.

- Ascites is the accumulation of fluid in the peritoneal cavity, causing abdominal swelling. In itself, this is an infection risk.
- Fluid transudates by discharging gradually through the pores in a membrane.
- Blood transfusion is the transfusion of blood or its components from one person to another.
- Hyperglycaemia is an excess of glucose in the bloodstream, often associated with diabetes mellitus. Hypoglycaemia is a deficiency of glucose in the bloodstream.
- Infection in the bloodstream is usually caused by bacteria getting into the bloodstream after a patient is given fluids intravenously, or receives a blood transfusion.
- Infections of the upper respiratory tract are usually minor, caused mostly by viruses, and commonly acquired in the community, for example influenza.
- A meatus is a passage or opening leading to the interior of the body, and therefore meatal cleansing entails cleansing of that opening.

INTRODUCTION

Currently, between 5 and 10% of patients admitted to acute care hospitals acquire one or more infections. Infection control is therefore a critical component of patient safety in South Africa. Identification of the risk factors can help to prevent the infections. Avoiding the use of invasive devices and using alternative strategies, as well as shortening the duration in which these devices are used, all work towards reducing the spread of nosocomial infections in our hospitals and health care services. The average hand-washing practice varied among hospitals from 16 to 81%. As we discussed in Chapter Two, barriers to compliance include understaffing, poor design of health care facilities, impractical guidelines and policies, and failure to apply behavioural change. A waterless alcohol-based hand-rub has been shown to be more practical than the standard hand-washing alone.

The four major problems in infection control in health care services, which we will address in this chapter, are:
1. urinary tract infection (catheter-associated), which is the most frequently contracted nosocomial infection (35%)
2. surgical site infection, which is the second most frequently contracted nosocomial infection (20%)
3. bloodstream infection, which is less commonly contracted (15%), but associated with high mortality and high costs, owing to the related use of an intravascular device

4. pneumonia (ventilator-associated), which is the least frequently contracted nosocomial infection (15%), and associated with high mortality rate (Burke 2007: 651–6).

A quarter of nosocomial infections involve patients in ICU, and nearly 70% are due to micro-organisms that are resistant to one or more antibiotics (Burke 2007: 651–6).

URINARY TRACT INFECTION (CATHETER-ASSOCIATED)

The normal bladder has several defences against infection, such as the difficulty of micro-organisms to pass along the urethra; the epithelial cells lining the bladder, which are resistant to bacterial adherence; and the process of urination, which ensures that bacteria do not manage to gain access to the bladder, are diluted by fresh urine and removed by the next urination. The presence of a urethral catheter interferes with these natural mechanisms. The urethral catheter is thus a major predisposing factor in urinary tract infections in health services (Wilson & Jenner 2007: 215).

A thorough understanding of the way in which biofilm forms on the surface of an indwelling catheter is central to the understanding of the pathogenesis of urinary tract infection. A biofilm is not a static, filmy slime layer, but rather a living organism composed of multiple species of bacteria and their secreted polysaccharide matrix, as well as components deposited from bodily fluids. The urinary catheter becomes encrusted with proteins, electrolytes and other organic molecules from the host's urine. Once a catheter has acquired a conditioning film, the features of the underlying catheter surface may be partially or completely obscured. The bare catheter surface is inhospitable to colonisation, but the conditioning film may encourage microbial attachment (Trautner & Darouiche 2004: 842–50). Trautner and Darouiche (2004: 843) propose that biofilms have two major effects:
1. They decrease susceptibility to anti-microbial agents.
2. They decrease susceptibility to microbiology laboratory results based on planktonic organisms in the bioflim.

Guidelines for insertion of urinary tract catheters

Urinary catheters should always be inserted at a minimum risk for infection. It is therefore safer to insert the catheter in the operating theatre, where the infection risk is lower. It is impossible to remove the perineal flora completely before catheterisation, and therefore the area should be cleaned with soap and water or saline. An antiseptic solution could also contribute to a reduction in urinary tract infections. The health care worker performing the procedure should be properly trained and competent. The catheter must be secured on the patient's leg to prevent movement in the urethra and discomfort for the patient.

A controlled trial by Burke et al. (1988), as described in (Wilson & Jenner 2007: 222), showed that catheterised patients who received no meatal cleansing had the lowest infection rate. Routine bathing or showering is all that is needed.

Prevention of urinary tract infection

The most frequent causative agents of nosocomial urinary tract infections are from the patients' colonic flora, or from health care personnel's hands, including *Escherichia coli*, enterococci, *Pseudomonas*, *Klebsiella*, enterobacter or candida (Trautner & Darouiche

The nine-point plan for handling catheter-associated urinary tract infection

1. Wash hands and use sterile gloves.
2. Prepare the patient, and position the patient comfortably.
3. Clean perineum and external meatus with saline, water and soap, or antiseptic agent, as per hospital policy.
4. Instil anaesthetic lubrication gel into the urethra.
5. Use sterile equipment.
6. Insert catheter directly into urethra.
7. Select catheter appropriately.
8. Inflate balloon with correct amount of sterile water.
9. Remove catheter as soon as possible.

Guidelines for maintaining the drainage system

1. Use a bag with an integral measuring chamber for patients on urine output monitoring.
2. Do not change the urine bag routinely.
3. Do not disconnect the catheter from the drainage bag, unless absolutely necessary.
4. Empty the bag as frequently as possible.
5. Wash hands before and after handling the drainage system.
6. Use clean gloves to handle the drainage system.
7. Empty urine into a clean container, and disinfect the container afterwards and wash your hands.
8. Take urine specimens from the sample port, not the drainage bag.
9. Ensure that the urine always flows downwards.
10. Avoid kinks in tubing.
11. Hang bag evenly on stand.
12. Do not change leg bag at night – connect it to an overnight drainage bag.
13. Avoid using bladder installations.

2004: 847). The difficulty in preventing these infections is compounded by catheter location, duration of the catheter *in situ*, and the number and types of organisms. The best way to prevent these infections is probably a closed drainage system, or intermittent catheterisation, ensuring dependent drainage and catheter removal when it is no longer needed. If possible, catheterisation could be avoided altogether. In the case of long-term catheterisation, clean, non-sterile, intermittent catheterisation has low rates of colonisation, that is, 20-40%. Urinary tract infections are lower when suprapubic catheters; condom catheters; or clean, non-sterile, intermittent catheters are used.

Nurses must ensure dependent drainage at all times, because a drainage tube that is below the level of the collection bag is associated with an increased risk of urinary tract infection. The need for the urinary tract catheter should often be reviewed in order to ensure that the catheter is removed as soon as possible. The following nine-point plan and guidelines for maintaining the drainage system will positively impact on the incidence of urinary tract infections in hospitals and health care services.

SURGICAL SITE INFECTION

Two thirds of surgical site infections are superficial and stem from bacterial inoculation during surgery. Interventions to decrease them after surgery have been shown to have little impact. There is a connection between the timing of anti-microbial administration and the effectiveness of antibiotics prophylaxis. Intra-operational anti-microbial administration with a high dose of antibiotics provides the best chance of avoiding infection. The longer the time lapses before the administration of antibiotics, the greater the chance of a surgical wound infection occurring. Four hours post-operation, for example, is too late to prevent the infection of a wound.

Surgical site infections may occur within the surgical site at any depth, starting from the skin itself and extending through the subcutaneous tissue, deep soft tissue (facia and muscle) into the deepest cavity of an organ.

Procedures involving sterile tissues, for example orthopaedic surgery, are likely to encounter little colonisation of bacteria and wound infections. By contrast, some parts of the body, for example the intestines, are colonised by large numbers of bacteria, which can enter the wound site while surgery is performed. In colon surgery, various methods are used to reduce the number of bacteria in the bowel. Surgery that involves a pre-existing infection or necrotic tissue is significantly more likely to result in surgical site infection.

The following procedures are listed in order of greatest susceptibility to infection to least susceptibility:
- limb amputation
- small bowel surgery
- large bowel surgery
- vascular surgery

- coronary bypass graft
- open reduction of long bone fractures
- hip prosthesis
- abdominal hysterectomy
- knee prosthesis.

Most surgical site infections are caused by gram-positive cocci, including *S. aureus*, *Staphylococcus epidermidis* and enterococcus. According to Cruse and Foord (1980), as described in Wilson & Jenner (2007: 182), the following are recognised measures for minimising the risk of surgical infections:

- A short preoperative hospital stay aims to prevent hospital organisms from colonising on the patient's skin.
- A preoperative disinfectant shower reduces the bacterial colonisation of the skin before the skin incision and therefore minimises the risk of infection.
- Alcohol solutions of iodine or chlorhexidine should be used to cleanse around the operation site.
- The skin should not be shaved.
- The wound should not become contaminated.
- Surgical technique should be meticulous.
- The operation time should be short.
- Scrupulous operation care should be given to the elderly, the obese, malnourished and diabetic patients.
- No drains must be brought out through the operation wound.
- The coagulation technique should be meticulous.
- Each surgeon should be kept informed of their wound infection rate as compared to that of their peers, as this can create awareness among medical staff and other staff members in the hospital.

The National Nosocomial Infections Surveillance System listed the factors below as the key elements in the development of surgical wound infections. Patients should be assessed for factors that can be corrected in the period preceding elective surgery. Open skin lesions should be allowed to heal and patients should be free from bacterial infections. The patient should also stop smoking, if possible, preferably one month before the surgery. Obese patients should try to lose some weight. The risk factors can be divided into the three categories, namely, patient, environmental and treatment factors.

Patient factors

The following host-derived factors are present in the patients at the time of the surgery and may contribute to surgical site infection. Ascites present in the patient prior to the operation could cause infection of the wound. Ascites is caused by transudation of fluid from the liver surface as a result of portal and lymphatic hypertension and increased membrane permeability, which leads to increased hydrostatic pressure and decreased oncotic pressure in the portal venous system. In itself this is an infection risk.

Chronic inflammation poses a risk to surgical wounds as the inflamed tissue could be a source of infection. Corticosteroid therapy is controversial in its ability to cause surgical site infection; it depresses the immune response and enables bacteria to multiply more easily in the wound.

Obesity poses a relative risk for surgical site infections because deep layers of adipose tissue can increase the complexity of the procedure and reduce the blood flow to the wound during healing.

Diabetes mellitus poses a relative risk among diabetic patients. The condition interferes with phagocytosis by white blood cells and causes a general increase in susceptibility to infection. The risk appears to be highest in insulin-dependent diabetes patients.

Extremes of age pose a risk because of the patient's immune response and other underlying diseases.

Hypocholesterolaemia, hypoxemia and peripheral vascular disease, with impairment of tissue oxygenation – such as may occur with vascular insufficiency or diabetes – will delay healing and thus increases the risk of wound infection.

Other, independent factors can also contribute to surgical site infections. These factors include prior site irradiation; recent operation; remote infection sites in the patient; skin carriage of staphylococci; skin disease in the area of infection (psoriasis), which can serve as a site for bacteria to colonise; under-nutrition, which causes delayed wound healing; and tobacco use, which can prevent sufficient oxygenation of the tissue.

Environmental factors

These factors can be present during and after a surgical procedure. The operation theatre must be controlled and checked for unsuitable equipment. Personal belongings should not be allowed in the room. Furthermore, contaminated and expired medication must be checked and discarded, and cleanliness must prevail.

The patient can prepare their skin preoperatively, by showering with an antibacterial soap the night before. The patient must not be shaved, as the risk of infection is increased by bacteria that colonise the inevitable small cuts and abrasions on the skin caused by shaving. The skin of the operation area must be cleaned with alcohol and needs to be completely dry before the incision is made. Special attention must be given to the navel with regard to cleaning and disinfection, as it can harbour bacteria, for example staphylococcus.

Peri-and intra-operative measures to prevent surgical site infections must be adhered to in hospitals. The preparation of the surgical team is also important – beards must be totally covered and masks must be handled carefully. The surgical team should focus on hand-washing procedures and should not operate with jewellery on their hands and arms. Movement in the theatre must be restricted. There should be no nailbrushes at the hand-wash basin as the scrubbing of nails, hands and arms opens up the scales of the skin, exposing the skin bacteria and thus contributing to surgical site infections. Moreover, brushes in a tray of antiseptic agent, like Savlon, can act as a biofilm and provide a breeding ground for bacteria.

Treatment factors

These factors can occur before, during and after surgery. Wound drains provide a route through which bacteria can enter the wound. However, a drain can also facilitate wound healing, by preventing the formation of haematomas. When a drain must be inserted during the operation, a closed drainage system should be used and a separate incision should be made for the drain, so that the main incision is not affected by the drain. Drains should not be left in place for too long, as this may enable bacteria to colonise the site. Emergency procedures, hypothermia, inadequate antibiotics prophylaxis and prolonged preoperative hospitalisation are all treatment factors that contribute to surgical wound infections.

Prolonged operating time creates a greater chance for bacteria to settle on the tissue or be carried from the hands or instruments to the wound. Although a wound infection can usually present itself 4 to 10 days after an operation, most of the infections have been introduced during surgery. As soon as the wound has been sutured, a loose mesh of fibrin is formed and is gradually infiltrated by fibroblasts and collagen. This structure becomes impervious to the entry of bacteria within a few hours, and with the theatre dressing in place for 48 hours undisturbed, pathogens are unlikely to gain access to the wound (Wilson & Jenner 2007: 182).

The post-operative period

Blood transfusion, and post-operative anaemia treated with a blood transfusion, are common and may be a life-saving act, but blood transfusions have been associated with increased rates of nosocomial infections following the penetration of the abdomen, with related factors such as shock or acute blood loss. According to Barie and Eachempati (2005: 1115–35), transfusion of any volume of red blood cells concentrates more than triple the risk of nosocomial infections, as compared to the case of no transfusions. Furthermore, observational studies have suggested that blood transfusion in critically ill patients may worsen organ dysfunction and increase mortality. An expanding body of evidence suggests that blood transfusion should be avoided as far as possible.

Hyperglycaemia, nutrition and blood sugar control have several effects on the host immune function. Hyperglycaemia may also be a marker of the catabolism and insulin resistance associated with surgical stress response. Poor control of blood glucose during surgery and in the peri-operative period increases the risk of infection, and thus worsens the outcome from sepsis. Ileus is common in critically ill surgical patients, and parenteral nutrition is used frequently for feeding, despite the poor efficacy and possible complications. Every effort should be made to provide enteral feeding, as it reduces the risk of nosocomial infections by more than half among critically ill patients (Barie & Eachempati 2005: 1128–9).

The administration of oxygen during the post-operative period can promote wound healing and prevent infection of the wound, but there are other, conflicting results, and more clinical trails need to be done in this regard (Barie & Eachempati 2005: 1129–30).

BLOODSTREAM INFECTION (IV DEVICE-ASSOCIATED)

Intravascular catheters are now an indispensable part of medical and nursing care. They are used to administer fluids, blood and nutritional support, and to perform haemodynamic monitoring of patients. The most significant infections associated with intravenous therapy are bloodstream infections; these contribute considerably to mortality among critically ill patients. The management of the IV catheter plays an important role in the incidence of nosocomial infections.

Guidelines for the insertion of an IV catheter are as follows:
- Wash hands before insertion.
- Use chlorhexidine to clean the skin and allow the skin to dry before insertion.
- Avoid shaving the skin.
- Secure catheter, but do not cover the insertion site with non-sterile tape.

Guidelines for the insertion of a central vascular catheter are as follows:
- Use a single lumen catheter, if possible.
- If catheter is needed for longer than 30 days, use a tunnelled or implantable device.
- Consider an anti-microbial impregnated device.
- Use optimal aseptic technique for insertion, with hand decontamination, sterile gloves and gowns, and large sterile drape.

Guidelines for the care of the insertion site are as follows:
- Wash hands before coming into contact with insertion site.
- Use sterile gauze or transparent film to cover the site.
- Change dressing only when it is no longer intact or when moisture collects at the site.
- Replace dressing at least every seven days.
- Clean site with aqueous chlorhexidine each time the dressing is changed.
- Inspect the site every two to three days for signs of infection (Wilson & Jenner 2007: 199–210).

Sepsis

Sepsis is infection in the bloodstream, usually caused by bacteria. There are always bacteria on the skin and on the surfaces of most objects. Thus health care providers clean the skin before they give an injection or IV fluids. They also wear gloves and use sterilised instruments and equipment to prevent the spread of bacteria and viruses.

A blood infection may occur when:
- the IV line is given through an infected area of skin
- there is a clot in the vein, which prevents the blood from flowing well
- an infection from one part of the body is spread to the injection site, or the catheter hub is contaminated by the patient's endogenous skin flora or by exogenous flora carried on the health care worker's hands
- the intravenous fluid is contaminated (Trautner & Darouiche 2004: 842).

Sepsis is more common in people whose immune systems are compromised owing to cancer treatment (radiation or chemotherapy), immune-suppressing drugs (for transplants or autoimmune diseases), chronic disease or immune-suppressing infections (such as HIV). Systemic inflammatory response syndrome (SIRS) is displayed by at least two of the following predisposing conditions:
- pulse rate of > 90/minute
- respiratory rate of 20 breaths/minute
- temperature of > 38 °C or < 35,5 °C
- a white blood cell count of > 12 000 or < 4 000/mm^3.

Sepsis is one of the most frequent causes of unplanned admission to the ICU. The pathophysiology of sepsis results from a complex interaction of cellular and inflammatory mediators. The release of these mediators represents the initiation of the host response to a pathogen. Then the synthesis of prostaglandins and activation of the complement and coagulation occurs. Under normal physiological conditions, pro-inflammatory mediators are moderated by anti-inflammatory cytokines. Failure of the body to control these mediators locally results in systemic overspill, which manifests as a general systemic inflammatory response. This exaggerated response, resulting in widespread cellular dysfunction, causes diverse physiological effects such as acute respiratory distress syndrome, disseminated intravascular coagulation and, eventually, multiple organ dysfunction syndrome (MODS). The term 'MODS' emphasises the range of severity in cases of multiple organ failure (Gupta & Jonas 2006: 143).

The organ dysfunction that characterises severe sepsis may include aspects such as circulatory failure secondary to septic shock, respiratory failure (PaO$_2$ FiO$_2$ < 26 kPa), renal failure with urine output of 0.5 ml/kg/hour despite fluid resuscitation, haematological failure and unexpected metabolic acidosis (lactate 0.4 mmol/l). Physiological effects of sepsis are tachypnoea, hypoxia, tachycardia, hypotension, lactic acidosis, oliguria, anuria with an increased level of creatinine, increased prothrombin time, increased activated partial thromboplastin time, failure to absorb feed, diarrhoea, jaundice, increased enzymes, low albumin and altered consciousness level (Gupta & Jonas 2006: 144).

Treatment priorities in severe sepsis include, among others, the following:
- Prompt recognition and early resuscitation.
- Appropriate antibiotic therapy after obtaining results from blood cultures.
- Source control, that is, the search for treatment of the focus of infection.
- Adjunct therapies, such as steroids and blood glucose control.
- Support for failing organs systems (Gupta & Jonas 2006: 144; Rivers, McIntyre, Morro & Rivers 2005: 1057–62).

Guidelines for treatment are as follows:
- A strategy of increased cardiac index to achieve an arbitrarily predefined elevated value is not recommended.
- High-dose corticosteroid therapy should not be used to treat septic shock.
- A weaning protocol should be in place, with spontaneous breathing trials.
- All patients should receive prophylaxis against deep venous thrombosis.
- All patients should receive prophylaxis against stress ulceration.

The Institute for Health Care Improvement promotes the use of care bundles to encourage change in current practice. A bundle is a group of evidence-based interventions related to a disease process, which, when carried out together, results in better patient outcomes. The sepsis care bundle is divided into a resuscitation bundle, which must be started immediately and completed within six hours of presentation of sepsis, and a management bundle, which should be implemented within 24 hours.

The sepsis resuscitation bundle comprises the following:
- Serum lactate measurement.
- Blood culture obtained before antibiotics are started.
- From the time of sepsis presentation, broad-spectrum antibiotic administration should start within three hours with regard to accident and emergency admissions, and within one hour in cases of non-accident and emergency ICU admissions.
- In the event of hypotension and/or lactate level greater than 4 mmol/l, crystalloid or the equivalent must be administered.
- Vasopressors should be applied for hypotension not responding to initial fluid resuscitation, to maintain a mean arterial pressure of above 65 mm Hg.

The sepsis management bundle comprises the following:
- Administration of low dose steroids.
- Administration of recombinant human-activated protein C.

- Glucose control maintained at less than 8.3 mmol/l.
- Inspiratory plateau pressure maintained at less than 30 cm H_2O in mechanically ventilated patients (Gupta & Jonas 2006: 145).

The cornerstone of the prevention of IV catheter-associated infections is infection control. Good hand hygiene, the use of maximal sterile barriers for catheter insertion and the use of specialised IV teams for catheter insertion and maintenance have all shown benefits.

PNEUMONIA (VENTILATOR-ASSOCIATED)

Occasionally, an upper respiratory tract infection may progress to a more serious infection of the lower respiratory tract, such as pneumonia. This could be life-threatening. Infection control and education remains the cornerstone in preventing nosocomial infection. A naso-gastric tube is associated with an increased risk of VAP as it may favour reflux of the gastric contents and enable micro-organisms to migrate to the upper airway. Enteral feeding may also increase microbial colonisation of the stomach by an elevated pH of the stomach and therefore provide a conducive environment for micro-organism growth.

The major risk factor for VAP is mechanically assisted ventilation, together with the underlying disease. Intubated patients are more likely to acquire VAP than are patients who are not intubated. Mucosa irritation and injury contribute to VAP because micro-organisms colonise the irritated areas. The nose filter is also bypassed, and intubation allows respiratory secretions to pool in the trachea above the cuff. The heavily contaminated secretions may leak around the cuff, particularly when it is deflated, or during suctioning procedures. Like all invasive tubing, endotracheal tubes are suspected of forming biofilms, which further add to the infection risk of intubated patients. Orotracheal intubation is associated with a lower risk for VAP.

Risk factors for post-operative pneumonia include the following:
- The type of surgery, such as abdominal aortic aneurysm repair, thoracic surgery, upper abdominal surgery.
- Emergency surgery.
- General anaesthetic.
- Transfusion of blood (more than four units).
- Critically ill patients.
- Age greater than 60 years.
- Impaired sensors.
- Chronic obstructive airway disease.
- Cerebrovascular accident.
- History of alcohol use.
- Smoking.

- Weight loss.
- Steroid use.
- Low or high blood urea nitrogen.

Contaminated respiratory equipment has frequently been incriminated in outbreaks because it can act as a reservoir and vehicle for the transmission of pathogens. Most of this equipment is in direct contact with mucous membranes, and therefore requires thorough cleaning and a high level of disinfection. Nebulisers and humidifiers should be decontaminated every 48 hours and always filled with sterile water. They should also always be changed between patient use and stored clean and dry (Cocanour, Peninger, Domonoske, et al. 2006: 122–8).

As listed in Table 5.1, certain non-pharmacological strategies have been evaluated for the prevention of VAP based on identified risk factors. The role of nursing is essential in many of these strategies.

CASE STUDY

Imagine that you are the sister-in-charge of a surgical ward in a local public hospital. On your ward round, you discover a patient with a wound infection. The surgical wound is red, and the patient's temperature is 38 °C. The patient is very tired and complains of pain in the wound area.

Questions

1. Identify the risk factors for a wound infection.
2. Describe the clinical presentation of the patient.
3. Explain how the risk for surgical site infection can be reduced.

Application to your own context

- How can you prevent surgical site infection in your ward?
- What is the procedure that should be followed when you find a patient with surgical site infection in the ward?

TIPS FOR NURSES

- Use aseptic procedures when you need to care for surgical wounds of patients, and when inserting a catheter.
- Wash hands with soap and water when hands are visibly dirty, or contaminated with bodily fluids.
- If hands are not visibly soiled, use an alcohol-based hand-rub for routine decontamination.
- Decontaminate hands before and after direct patient contact.
- Decontaminate hands after removing gloves and comply with standard hand hygiene protocol of the health organisation.

Table 5.1 Strategies for the prevention of VAP

Number	Strategy	Efficacy
1	Use of protective gowns and gloves	Proven
2	Provision of adequate nutritional support	Proven
3	Dedicated use of disposable suction catheters	Unproven
4	Adequate hand-washing between patient contacts	Proven
5	Maintenance of adequate pressure in endotracheal tube cuff	Proven
6	Chest physiotherapy	Unproven
7	Avoidance of gastric over-distension	Proven
8	Removal of nasogastric tube as soon as is clinically feasible	Proven
9	Humification with heat and moisture exchanges	Proven
10	Routine changes of ventilator circuit	Unproven
11	Postural changes	Proven
12	Humification with heat and moisture exchanges with bacterial filter	Unproven
13	Semi-recumbent positioning of patient	Proven
14	Daily changes of heat and moisture exchanges	Unproven
15	Chlorhexidine oral rinse	Proven
16	Use of a formal infection control programme	Proven
17	Routine changes of in-line catheter	Unproven
18	Scheduled drainage of condensate from ventilator circuits	Proven
19	Continuous subglottic suctioning	Proven

Source: Cocanour, Peninger, Domonoske, *et al.* (2006: 122–8); Ricart, Lorente, Diaz, *et al.* (2003: 2695)

- Surgical hand antisepsis using an anti-microbial soap or an alcohol-based hand-rub with persistent activity is recommended before sterile gloves are put on (Ziady & Small 2004: 178).

PRECAUTIONS

Particular diligence regarding prescriptions is essential in the prevention of infection. Always ask if you are not sure about a procedure. Ensure the correct procedure when inserting a urinary tract catheter. Pay meticulous attention to hand-washing and gloving before an aseptic procedure. Pay attention also to the drainage system, and do not interrupt the aseptic technique when handling a patient with a urinary tract catheter. Implement strategies for surgical patients that prevent nosocomial infections, such as short preoperative hospital stay, disinfection shower pre-op, avoidance of shaving of the skin and avoidance of wound contamination. Implement meticulous surgical technique. Prevent bloodstream infections by complying with the guidelines for insertion of IV catheters. Acquaint yourself with SIRS by being alert to the predisposing conditions. Always apply infection control measures to prevent VAP infections, especially if the patient is mechanically ventilated.

CONCLUSION

Behavioural change remains the biggest obstacle – cross-infection of patients by health care workers with contaminated hands is still a major source of infection in health care services.

SELF-ASSESSMENT

Before moving on to the next chapter, make sure that you can discuss the following key concepts and their application in your context with a colleague:

- Risk factors for VAP.
- Explain how you would ensure aseptic technique for your patient when inserting an IV device.

FURTHER READING AND WEB RESOURCES

http://www.cdc.gov/ncidod/hip
http://www.med.upenn.edu
http://www.hopisafe.ch

CHAPTER SIX

African haemorrhagic fevers

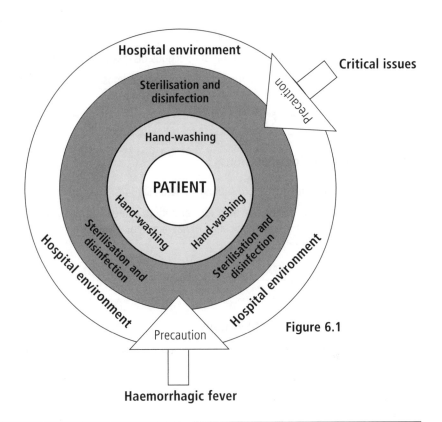

Figure 6.1

Haemorrhagic fever

Learning outcomes

Upon completion of this chapter, you should be able to:

- identify signs and symptoms of the African haemorrhagic fevers, such as Lassa fever, Rift Valley fever, Congo-Crimea fever, Ebola and Marburg fever, and yellow fever
- describe the correct precautions and procedures for caring for a patient with haemorrhagic fever.

Learning assumed to be in place

To gain the most benefit from this chapter, you should already have the following knowledge and skills:

- Knowledge of basic effective hygiene.
- Knowledge of aseptic procedures.
- Knowledge of the prevention of infectious diseases in a hospital.
- Knowledge of sterilisation and disinfection methods.

Key ethical considerations

- Health professionals are sharing vulnerability in cases of haemorrhagic fever.
- Nurses and doctors have an ethical duty to protect themselves and other health care users against amplification of haemorrhagic fever by complying with standard precautions.

Key legislative considerations

All suspected cases of haemorrhagic fever must be notified to the local officer for infectious diseases at the designated authority.

Important terms

Haemorrhagic fever is caused by four families of causative viruses, as shown in Table 6.1. Lassa fever is caused by Lassa virus. Rift Valley fever, caused by the Bunyaviridae phlebovirus, was first reported with mosquitoes as the vectors. The severe Congo-Crimea haemorrhagic fever is caused by the Bunyaviridae nairovirus. The reservoir of the Ebola virus is unknown. Yellow fever occurs in monkeys that are infected by mosquitoes.

INTRODUCTION

Haemorrhagic fever is caused by four families of causative viruses, as shown in Table 6.1. While members of each family share many common features in their pathogenesis, there are significant differences between families and genera (Peters, Sherrif & Zaki 2002: 268). The viruses are small RNA viruses believed to have aerosol infectivity and cause disease during the period of viremia, or acute illness.

Table 6.1 Viral haemorrhagic fevers

Virus	Related haemorrhagic fever
Arenaviridae	Lassa and South American haemorrhagic fever
Bunyaviridae: • Phlebovirus • Nairovirus • Hantavirus	Rift Valley fever Congo-Crimea haemorrhagic fever Haemorrhagic fever with renal syndrome and Hantavirus pulmonary syndrome
Filoviridae filovirus	Ebola and Marburg
Flavivirus	Yellow fever

Some of the haemorrhagic fever viruses have almost no cytopathic effects, whereas others are highly deconstructive of the cells they infect. Disseminated intravascular coagulation (DIC) occurs in some, but not all. Involvement of the liver also varies. Most of these fevers are worst while the virus is actively replicating in the organs. There is now considerable information available that suggests that immune enhancement and immunopathology are the major factors in the genesis of the syndrome of haemorrhagic fever.

ARENAVIRIDAE – LASSA FEVER

Lassa fever is caused by the Lassa virus (LV), a member of the family Arenaviridae, which maintains itself as a lifelong infection of a rodent host, *Mastomys natalensis*, in which it is mostly inactive. This rodent is well adapted to peridomestic life in West African villages. Accidental human exposure to the virus is therefore frequent. Lassa fever is ever present and likely to increase in Africa, as so many larger communities in West Africa are affected and the threat to visitors and relief workers in rural areas grows. Several deaths have occurred, owing to lack of awareness of these risks and a delay in diagnosis.

Lassa fever is treatable with ribavirin, the earlier the more effective. Household and sexual contact with persons ill, or recently ill, with Lassa is a significant risk factor for human-to-human transmission. Nosocomial transmission to hospital staff or other patients has also been recorded and may be prevented through the use of simple standard precautions and barrier nursing principles. Hospital outbreaks of Lassa fever have been associated with:

- inadequate disinfection
- ill-advised surgery on patients with abdominal pain and fever
- direct contact with blood and contaminated needles
- indiscriminate use of needles for intravenous therapy
- injections with inadequate needle and syringe sterilisation (Fisher-Hoch 2005: 123–37; Richmond & Bagolbe 2003: 1271–5).

The disease begins with the onset of fever and non-specific symptoms such as headache, generalised weakness and malaise. This is followed within days by sore throat, retrosternal pain, conjunctival infection, abdominal pain and diarrhoea. Severe cases may then progress to facial and neck swelling, bleeding, shock and multi-organ system failure. Mortality estimates range from 2% in community-based studies to as high as 50% in nosocomial outbreaks. Patients with the following signs and symptoms should be treated as highly suspected of Lassa fever, especially when they came from Africa or have visited an African country:

- Severe fever (haemorrhagic) in an adult.
- Diarrhoea and vomiting, abdominal pain and dysphasia.
- Pulmonary and chest pain with coughing.
- Oedema.
- Neurological signs like headache and meningitis.
- Conjunctivitis.
- Sore, inflamed pharynx or larynx.
- Arthralgia (joint pain) and back pain.
- Hepatic dysfunction and proteinuria (Fisher-Hoch 2005: 123–37).

BUNYAVIRIDAE (PHLEBOVIRUS) – RIFT VALLEY FEVER

Rift Valley fever (RVF) is caused by the Bunyaviridae Phlebovirus, and is primarily a mosquito-borne viral disease. The reservoir is almost certainly sheep and cattle, but can also be aerosols generated from bodily fluids and the tissues of diseased animals. Person-to-person transmission has not been reported. There is an incubation period of three to five days and the diagnosis can be made through diagnostic tests such as viral blood culture and cerebrospinal fluid.

The onset is sudden, with chills, myalgia, joint pains, headache and a biphasic fever that lasts about a week. Patients often complain of nausea, vomiting, and abdominal fullness and pain. There is bradycardia, with slight tenderness over the liver, which may be enlarged. Patients can become delirious and have hallucinations.

RVF is unique in having a highly variable clinical presentation that includes viral haemorrhagic fever, encephalitis, optic neuropathy resulting in retinal disease, and hepatitis. The late onset of the interferon (IFN) response is associated with more severe diseases, such as DIC, microangiopathic haemolytic anaemia and intravascular deposition of fibrin thrombi. The delay in IFN-alpha response is to allow more extensive infection of vascular endothelium. The virus causes rapid cell death in all mammalian cells (Peters, Sherrif & Zaki 2002: 270). Death usually follows massive gastrointestinal haemorrhage, oliguria, anuria and acute renal failure after three to six days (Goad & Nguyen 2003: 69). Animal studies suggest a possible role for ribavirin medication.

RVF was first reported in West Africa in 1974, carried by mosquitoes in Senegal. However, large outbreaks in the area were then not reported prior to an epidemic in southern Mauritania in 1987. The first outbreak outside of sub-Saharan Africa occurred in Egypt in 1977. From 1974 to 1976, an outbreak was reported in South Africa. Epizootics of RVF are usually associated with years of unusually heavy rainfall and localised flooding. Pools of standing water promote excessive mosquito numbers, which can infect livestock. The disease usually occurs first in animals, then in humans. Human infection occurs mainly among farmers and others at occupational risk. Bats infected with RVF have been identified in Guinea (CDC 2002: 2989–90).

BUNYAVIRIDAE (NAIROVIRUS) – CONGO-CRIMEA FEVER

Congo-Crimea haemorrhagic fever is severe and caused by the Bunyaviridae Nairovirus. The reservoirs are hare, bird, ticks, cattle, sheep, goats and ostrich, with the vector being ticks and the vehicle being infected secretions from patients or livestock. The virus has been found among ticks in Africa, Asia, the Middle East and eastern Europe. The virus is transmitted to humans through the bites of ticks (hyalomma) or contact with infected livestock blood and tissues. Human-to-human transmission can also occur.

The incubation period is one to six days, and diagnosis can be made through diagnostic tests such as viral blood culture, cerebrospinal fluid (CSF) and tissue. The patient can present with headache, chills, myalgia, abdominal pain, photophobia, petechiae, thrombocytopaenia and leukopaenia, conjunctivitis and pharyngitis three to seven days after being bitten by a tick.

Later, the patient may experience sharp mood swings, and may become confused and aggressive. After two to four days, agitation can be replaced by depression and lassitude, and abdominal pain may localise to the right upper quadrant, with detectable hepatomegaly. Other clinical signs at this stage include tachycardia, lymphadenopathy and a petechial rash, which progresses to ecchymosis and other bleeding. There is usually evidence of hepatitis. The severely ill may develop hepatorenal and pulmonary failure after the fifth day of illness. The mortality rate is approximately 30%, with death occurring in the second week of illness. Patients must be treated with isolation and supportive therapy with ribavirin. In the patients who recover, improvement generally begins on the ninth or tenth day after onset of illness.

FILOVIRIDAE FILOVIRUS – EBOLA AND MARBURG FEVER

Four strains of the Ebola virus have been described, as Ivory Coast, Reston, Sudan and Zaire strains. The reservoir is unknown, but it could be a primate, guinea pig or bat, with no vector. The vehicle is infected secretions, and in health services it is the contact needle or syringe that has been re-used without proper disinfection.

The incubation period is 5 to12 days, and diagnosis can be made through a diagnostic test such as blood culture. The patient usually presents clinically with fever, myalgia, arthralgia, sore throat, vomiting, diarrhoea, abdominal pain, conjunctivitis, hepatic dysfunction and maculopapular rash. Dehydration and significant wasting occur as the disease progresses. Later, the central nervous system frequently becomes involved, manifested by delirium, or coma. The patient must be nursed in strict isolation.

The symptoms and signs of the Marburg and Ebola virus infections are similar (Ndayimirije & Kay 2005: 2155–7).

Typically, there is evidence of an outbreak or case cluster of possible Ebola virus and the patient is either 60 years old or more, or a child of less than two years, presenting with the above-mentioned severe clinical features and is hospitalised with query haemorrhagic fever, or with Aids.

The legacy of years of poverty has led to extremely poor medical education and services in most parts of Africa, which provides the conditions for the spread of Marburg haemorrhagic fever in medical facilities. The high mortality rate of the fever in Africa may also be related to parenteral exposure, and particularly needle exposure in clinics through vaccine administration and use of multidose vials. Prevention of future outbreaks will not be easy. Technically, vaccines for all the haemorrhagic diseases can be made, but funding for development and delivery costs must first become available. Moreover, it is difficult to identify exposed populations in Africa, and even harder to reach them (Fisher-Hoch 2005: 134–5).

What rather needs to be done is to concentrate on disseminating and implementing an understanding of blood-borne virus risks, and on practising the disciplines of effective training and clinical practice. Training of medical and other health professionals is a critical component in preventing the spread of further infections. When health professionals are better trained and informed about preventative measures and infection control strategies, hospital personnel, patients and their families in endemic areas and referral hospitals can be better protected. Education of the public and the consumer is also a powerful tool in the prevention of an outbreak of Marburg fever.

Community members must insist on new needles and syringes when health care is offered to them. They should preferably buy their own needles and syringes, as in parts of Africa health professionals re-use needles and syringes and unwittingly add to the spread and amplification of Ebola and Marburg fever at the health care facilities. Public health care providers must remember that poor people are undereducated, and not stupid. Patients and community members learn quickly that the hospital is the place where people become infected with viral haemorrhagic fevers, and in reaction they desert the hospital and even hide their sickness from medical personnel. Although these actions make case-finding difficult, they have been the most frequent and effective means by which filovirus outbreaks have been terminated (Fisher-Hoch 2005: 135; Richards, Murphy, Reeve, *et al.* 2000: 240–4).

FLAVIVIRUS – YELLOW FEVER

Yellow fever is a mosquito-borne infection endemic to non-urban areas of tropical South America and sub-Saharan Africa. Up to 50% of haemorrhagic fever-related mortality can be attributed to this fever. Immunisation campaigns gradually eradicated yellow fever in some countries, and in Africa control programmes slackened and the disease began to recur from time to time.

Clinical features of yellow fever are abrupt after a three- to six-day incubation period. They include flu-like symptoms, such as fever, chills, malaise, headache, myalgia, nausea and dizziness. There are three phases:
1. Sudden infection and onset of flu-like symptoms, with bradycardia.
2. A remission phase, lasting 24 hours, before the symptoms return.
3. An intoxication phase, characterised by jaundice, albuminuria, oliguria, cardiovascular instability and haemorrhagic manifestations.

Death occurs usually around 7 to 10 days of ongoing liver failure and metabolic acidosis (Isaacson 2001: 1707–12).

Table 6.2 on pages 68 to 69 summarises the main points of these four African haemorrhagic fevers.

CASE STUDY

A 38-year-old businessman from New York died after travelling from January to March in West Africa to take care of his crops and an infestation of multi-mammate rats. The patient was born in Liberia and had resided in the USA for five years. The onset of his illness included fever, chills, severe sore throat, diarrhoea and back pain. He travelled by airplane through London before arriving in New York, and then he travelled by train to his home. Within hours of reaching home, he was hospitalised and treated for malaria and typhoid fever. His condition deteriorated, and the CDC and Department of Health were notified. The patient died before the virus or organism could be identified.

Questions

1. Identify and describe the disease.
2. Identify the medication that you would have given to the patient.
3. Outline your investigation methods of identifying possible persons who came into contact with the patient. Also state how you would handle the contacts.
4. Where does this disease usually amplify?

Table 6.2 Characteristics of African haemorrhagic fevers

Haemorrhagic fever	Location	Diagnosis	Cause	Effect	Symptoms	Treatment
Lassa	West Africa	Sudden onset with severe fever and chills, diarrhea and vomiting, chest pain, edema, head ache, conjunctivitis, back pain and a history of visiting or living in West Africa and working with sheep and cattle	Lassa virus, Arenaviridae	Mortality estimates: 2% in community-based studies, 50% in nosocomial outbreaks	Onset of fever, non-specific symptoms such as headache, generalised weakness and malaise, followed by sore throat, retrosternal pain, conjunctival infection, abdominal pain and diarrhoea; then possibly facial and neck swelling, bleeding, shock and multi-organ system failure	Ribavirin
Rift Valley	West Africa, southern Mauritania, Egypt, South Africa	Incubation period of 3–5 days; diagnosis made through viral blood culture and cerebrospinal fluid tests	Mosquito-borne Bunyaviridae phlebovirus; reservoirs are sheep and cattle, or aerosols from bodily fluids and diseased animal tissue	Massive gastrointestinal haemorrhage, oliguria, anuria and acute renal failure	Sudden onset of chills, myalgia, joint pains, headache and biphasic fever; nausea, vomiting, and abdominal fullness and pain; bradycardia, possibly enlarged liver; delirium and hallucinations; highly variable clinical presentation including viral haemorrhagic fever, encephalitis, optic neuropathy and hepatitis	Possibly Ribavirin
Congo-Crimea	Africa, Asia, the Middle East, eastern Europe	Incubation period of 1–6 days; diagnosis made through viral blood culture, and cerebrospinal fluid and tissue tests	Bunyaviridae nairovirus; reservoirs are hare, bird, ticks, cattle, sheep, goats, ostrich; vector is ticks; vehicle is infected secretions	Mortality rate of about 30%, with death occurring in the second week; in patients who recover, improvement begins 9 or 10 days after onset of illness	Headache, chills, myalgia, abdominal pain, photophobia, petechiae, thrombocytopaenia and leukopaenia, conjunctivitis and pharyngitis; sharp mood swings, confusion and aggression; depression, lassitude; abdominal pain may localise to the right upper quadrant; tachycardia, lymphadenopathy, petechial rash progressing to ecchymosis and other bleeding; hepatitis; hepatorenal and pulmonary failure	Isolation, Ribavirin supportive therapy

Ebola and Marburg	Ivory Coast, Reston, Sudan and Zaire	Incubation period of 5–12 days; diagnosis made through blood culture	*Ebola* – reservoir unknown, possibly primate, guinea pig or bat; no vector; vehicle is infected secretions or contact needle or syringe	Mortality rate of 50–90% with amplification in health services involving multiple uses of needles and multidose vials	Fever, myalgia, arthralgia, sore throat, vomiting, diarrhoea, abdominal pain, conjunctivitis, hepatic dysfunction, maculopapular rash; dehydration, significant wasting; delirium or coma	Strict isolation
Yellow fever	Non-urban areas of tropical South America and sub-Saharan Africa	Incubation period of 3–6 days	Mosquito-borne Flavivirus	Responsible for up to 50% haemorrhagic fever-related mortality	Death follows 7–10 days of ongoing liver failure and metabolic acidosis. Fever, chills, malaise, headache, myalgia, nausea, dizziness; sudden infection and onset of flu-like symptoms, with bradycardia; brief remission; jaundice, albuminuria, oliguria, cardiovascular instability and haemorrhagic manifestations	No specific treatment available. Give support and admit patient to intensive care unit if patient is very sick.

Application to your own context

- Ensure that you and your nursing team know how to nurse patients with haemorrhagic diseases.
- Study several case studies on care of patients with haemorrhagic diseases, and ask questions regarding the nursing care and precautions that were implemented.

TIPS FOR NURSES

To ensure safe practices in health care facilities, health care professionals must always be on the alert for haemorrhagic diseases, especially if patients come from or have just visited another country.

PRECAUTIONS

One cannot plead ignorance – haemorrhagic fevers are classified as dangerous pathogens! Always apply standard precautions with all patients entering the health services. At confirmation of a haemorrhagic disease, strict isolation precautions must be instituted. Movement of the patient should not be allowed. The absolute minimum of staff should have contact with the patient, for example one nurse and one doctor. Nothing should be removed from the room. Appropriate protective clothing should be worn as per infection control standards. Disposable equipment and a hypochlorite solution for cleaning should all be used, and all waste should be treated as clinical waste.

CONCLUSION

Increasingly, international travel has resulted in the importation of microbial agents not endemic to South Africa and its neighbouring countries. This poses diagnostic challenges to health care providers, and careful assessment of any travelling to regions where uncommon diseases are endemic should be addressed and noted. In non-endemic areas, health care professionals must identify a haemorrhagic fever by enquiring about the travel history of the patient, the incubation period and the common clinical signs and symptoms of these diseases. The common presentations are fever, myalgias, petechiae and shock. Health care professionals should always be aware of the potential risk of tropical viral haemorrhagic fevers in order to ensure a correct and proper diagnosis, followed by rapid management of the patient and minimisation of the chances of nosocomial infections, where the disease can amplify in the hospital.

SELF-ASSESSMENT

Before moving on to the next chapter, make sure that you can discuss the following key concepts and their application in your context with a colleague:

- The precautions that health care professionals should take to prevent haemorrhagic fever from amplifying.
- Identify the main features of haemorrhagic fevers.

FURTHER READING AND WEB RESOURCES

http://www.who.int/emc/diseases/ebola/index.html
http://www.cdc.gov/ncidod/diseases/list_mosquitoborne.htm
http://www.cdc.gov/ncidod/dvbid/yellowfever/index.htm
http://www.who.int/emc/diseases/ebola/index.html
http://www.cdc.gov/ncidod/diseases/list_mosquitoborne.htm
http://www.who.int/emc/diseases/ebola/index.html
http://www.who.int/csr/disease/ebola/en/   http://www.cdc.gov/ncidod/dvrd/spb/mnpages/dispages/arena.htm http://www.who.int/emc/diseases/ebola/index.html
http://www.cdc.gov/ncidod/diseases/virlfvr/virlfvr.htm

CHAPTER SEVEN

Emerging infections

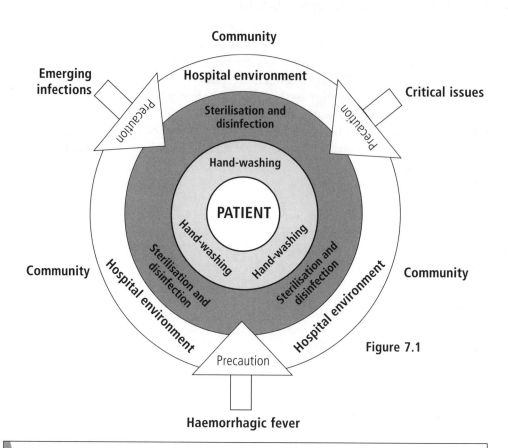

Figure 7.1

Learning outcomes

Upon completion of this chapter, you should be able to:

- explain these diseases: avian flu, multiple drug-resistant tuberculosis (MDR TB), extremely drug-resistant tuberculosis (XDR TB), severe acute respiratory syndrome (SARS) and human immunodeficiency virus (HIV)
- identify infection control measures for these infectious diseases.

Learning assumed to be in place

To gain the most benefit from this chapter, you should already have the following knowledge and skills:

- Basic knowledge of TB, avian flu, SARS, and HIV and Aids.
- Knowledge of basic effective hygiene.
- Knowledge of aseptic procedures.
- Knowledge of the prevention of infectious diseases in a hospital.
- Knowledge of sterilisation and disinfection methods.

Key ethical considerations

Health professionals have a duty to ensure, when dealing with patients who have infectious diseases, that they prevent the spread of the disease and thereby protect themselves and their colleagues and other patients.

Key legislative considerations

- By law, certain conditions have been classified as legally modifiable, some owing to their risk of infection transmission and some with the aim of evaluating the health status of communities.
- The list of conditions is periodically updated and published by the Minister of Health in the *Government Gazette*. This process of notification must be done on the GW 17/5 form, according to the *National Health Act (61 of 2003)*.

Important terms

- Avian flu, or bird flu, is known to be of animal origin and has caused infection in humans.
- Multiple drug-resistant TB is self-evidently multi-drug-resistant, while extremely drug-resistant TB resists isoniazid and rifampicin.
- Severe acute respiratory syndrome recently emerged as a severe respiratory infection.
- Sexual contact is the primary method of HIV transmission in the world.

INTRODUCTION

Some diseases lie dormant and then emerge periodically, at times as a stronger virus, with more resistance to modern medication. Health care personnel should always be on the lookout for these diseases.

AVIAN FLU

'This is a frightening disease. ICU admission is needed in 23% of patients, and the mortality rate is 14% of those admitted. Soon, ICU facilities will be overwhelmed and there will be a rapid rise in mortality.' (Richards 2007)

Avian flu, H5N1, is a novel, or new, virus, crossing the species barrier with virulent infection, and is efficiently transmitted from human to human. The H5N1 was first described in birds in China. Treatment of the virus posed a problem, as the circulating birds were difficult to get rid of and culling them did not remove the virus. The virus spread to humans because of the high density in the poultry and human populations.

Persons vulnerable to avian flu are those who smoke and have contact with poultry. Lung X-rays of patients were shown to be abnormal on admission and infiltrated. Infected people tend to present with a fever of > 38 °C, and the flu-like symptoms of headaches, myalgias, sore throat and rhinitis. Respiratory symptoms such as cough and dyspnoea are common. Gastrointestinal symptoms such as diarrhoea, vomiting and abdominal pain are also associated. The mortality rate is high, and most patients die of progressive respiratory failure and multiple organ dysfunction. For treatment, most patients require mechanical ventilation and broad-spectrum antibiotics.

All persons travelling to areas of H5N1 infection should ensure that their vaccinations are up to date; they should also visit the CDC website for the latest information (www.cdc.gov). A medical travel kit should be prepared with a thermometer and alcohol-based hand-rub. The CDC also recommends that travellers should avoid poultry and that all poultry-related foods should be treated with caution, for example eggs should be well cooked. As always, aggressive and frequent hand-washing is advised.

Only persons with a travel history to the involved area are at risk. Exposed people should be quarantined at home, as the spread occurs in hospitals. Infection control precautions for hospital staff are basic, and staff should shower on leaving the premises, wear a surgical mask (N95) that fits properly, wash their hands frequently, and avoid touching their eyes, nose and mouth as well as other people. They should always wear gowns and caps of impermeable material, gloves at all times in the ICU, and eye protection when dealing with possibly infected patients. When the patient is ventilated, staff should avoid nebulisers and use Hudson masks and closed-system suctioning. Contaminated surfaces should be disinfected with household bleach.

There are three phases in preparing for an influenza pandemic:

1. **The pre-event phase:** The objective is to ensure preparedness for a potential outbreak through training, communication, surveillance, infection control and vaccination. Effective pre-event risk communication is known to reduce risk during the event phase – the purpose of initiating training and communication at this stage is to enhance decision-making capabilities when the pandemic actually occurs. The non-specific nature of the initial manifestations of H5N1 infection in humans confounds case detection.

    Knowing how H5N1 infection is transmitted is important for infection control in this phase. The route from avian flu-infected patients to health care workers is uncertain, but inhalation of infectious respiratory secretions, or contact with virus-laden secretions, is thought to be responsible. Although the current routine flu vaccines are not likely to protect against a pandemic strain of influenza, vaccination against seasonal influenza should be actively promoted in people most likely to come into contact with a pandemic strain, such as all health care workers. During the pre-event phase, the main objectives are to reduce opportunities for human infection and to strengthen the early warning system for the disease.

2. **The event phase:** Once the wide-scale outbreak is declared, an event phase comes into being. The aim is to implement effective measures to ensure a rapid and appropriate response. Advanced planning is important, based on principles of leadership, communication, surveillance, capacity management and support.

3. **The post-event phase:** During this phase, the effects of the pandemic and the extent to which the core functions have been disrupted are measured. The main objective is to contain or delay the spread at the source.

    During this phase, remedial measures need to be taken to restore the core functions. Vigilance in preparation for subsequent waves of the pandemic should be maintained. Psychosocial support should continue for staff and other health care professionals. Morbidity, mortality and social disruption should be reduced as much as possible, and research should be conducted to guide response measures (Tiwari, Tarrant, Yuen, *et al.* 2006: 308–13; WHO 2006: 1–4).

SEVERE ACUTE RESPIRATORY SYNDROME

SARS is a severe pneumonic disease caused by a corona virus, SAR-CoV. It was first recognised in November 2002 in the Guangdong province, China, and by July of the next year it had spread to 32 countries and affected more than 800 people. The virus had been found in a number of wild animals, and contact with these animals could have been the origin of the infection in humans.

The infection is associated with considerable morbidity, with an average case fatality of 15%. Death is highest in older persons and those with co-morbidities. Children are rarely affected. The primary mode of infection appears to be direct contact between infectious respiratory secretions and mucous membranes, such as in the eyes, mouth and nose. Transmission may occur through contact with bodily fluids at these sites and contaminated fomites, but evidence showing this is limited. The incubation period is four to six days, and patients are most infectious on the tenth day. Infection and transmission occur in most cases in hospitals where the disease amplifies, as well as during high-risk procedures that cause aerosolisation of respiratory secretions, such as intubation and suctioning.

Early identification of cases, and vigorous contact tracing and home quarantine of close contacts during the incubation period, is important in prevention of outbreaks of SARS (Wilson & Jenner 2007: 238–9).

MULTIPLE DRUG-RESISTANT TB AND EXTREMELY DRUG-RESISTANT TB

Mycobacteria are gram-positive bacteria characterised by unusual staining properties. They are termed 'acid-fast bacilli' (AFB) because, unlike most bacteria, their cell walls retain the stain after treatment with strong acids. There are many species. The human pathogens are *M. TB* and *M. leprae*, which cause TB and leprosy respectively. The usual site of infection is the lungs, where pulmonary TB occurs (Wilson & Jenner 2007: 125).

MDR TB is essentially a human-made problem. In most cases, it emerges when a TB patient receives inappropriate or ineffective treatment, which allows naturally resistant TB bacteria to survive and multiply (Weyer, Van der Walt & Kantor 2006: 1). It is a new emergent strain that seems to resist nearly every existing drug. Already present on every continent, a recent outbreak in South Africa proved of particular concern because of its extraordinarily virulent form combined with the fact that it occurred in a region of extremely high HIV and Aids co-infection. The WHO said that multi-drug-resistant strains are mainly owing to health care workers' improper treatment regimes and failure to ensure that patients complete the course of treatment. The task team of the WHO developed a seven-point plan of action on this TB:

The MDR TB seven-point plan of action

1. Conduct rapid surveys of the strain.
2. Enhance laboratory capacity.
3. Improve technical capacity of clinical and public health managers to effectively respond to outbreaks.
4. Implement infection control precautions.
5. Increase research support for the development of anti-TB drugs.
6. Increase research support for TB.
7. Promote universal access to antiretroviral drugs (Moszynski 2006: 566).

The side-effects of MDR TB are severe. Patients who default on their treatment and those whose treatment fails become chronic MDR TB carriers and pose a significant threat to public health.

XDR TB stems from poor general TB control and the consequent development of MDR TB and is associated with high mortality rates. HIV-infected patients are particular vulnerable. Treatment is difficult, and appropriate second-line drugs are not universally available. XDR TB resists rifampicin and isoniazid.

Infection control measures should be implemented rapidly in health care organisations and other high-risk areas, such as prisons, in order for transmission of these types of TB to be reduced.

HIV AND AIDS

The exact HIV seroprevalence rates among patients in South African hospitals are not known. However, there are a few factors that need to be considered here. The numbers of HIV and Aids patients in our hospitals are increasing. Currently, hospitals are catering for higher levels of acuity in patients, and in a shorter time span. HIV-positive patients are more likely to have nosocomial infections than are HIV-negative patients, by virtue of their treatment, such as long-term, antiretroviral drug administration. Contamination of water supplies also adds to the problem. Furthermore, contamination of the hospital environment by organisms such as *C. difficile*, *Cryptosporidium parvum* and *Mycobacterium avium* complex pose a particular hazard to the HIV-positive patient (Duse 1999: 193). Because of these risks, efforts should be made to understand specific risk factors, and control measures should be implemented in health care institutions.

Nosocomial TB in HIV-positive patients poses the risk of active TB with an accelerated course (Laing 1999: 180). The spread of MDR TB between HIV-positive patients is a serious concern. The delay in recognition of MDR TB, and therefore the delayed initiation of effective drug therapy and poor infection control measures, are major factors in the spread of nosocomial MDR TB. Research studies (Striud, Tokars & Grieco 1995; Wenger, Otten, Breeden, *et al.* 1995, as cited in Laing 1999: 180) indicated that the best way of preventing TB among patients and health care workers is the introduction of strict isolation facilities in negative pressure rooms until the patient is found to be negative for at least three sputum samples. In addition, it was stated that nebulised therapy and physiotherapy should be conducted in adapted respiratory isolation rooms that allow sufficient air changes to remove possible airborne particles.

Furthermore, an American study (Bouza, Blazquez, Rodriques-Creixems, *et al.* 1996, as cited in Laing 1999: 180–1), reported gram-negative nosocomial pneumonias, with organisms such as *Klebsiella*, *Enterobacter* and *Pseudomonas*, in HIV-positive patients who died within a week of diagnosis (Laing 1999: 181). Another study (Goetz, Squier, Wagener & Mulder 1994, as cited in Laing 1999: 81) pointed out that *S. aureus*, *Streptococcus pneumonia*, *Haemophilus influenzae* and *Viridans streptococci* are among the pathogens that cause nosocomial infections in HIV-positive patients.

Pseudomonas infection in HIV-positive patients is most commonly found in the lungs and tends to occur in the hospital environment, according to one study (Bouza, Blazquez, Rodriques-Creixems, *et al.* 1996, as cited in Laing 1999: 181). Another nosocomial infection is the transmission from Aids patients to cancer patients, which has been suggested as a possible explanation for the rise of *Pneumocystis carinii pneumonia*, reported among cancer patients after the onset of the Aids pandemic.

Certain studies (Frank, Daschne, Schulgen & Milss 1997, as cited in Padoveze, Trabasso & Branchini 2002: 347) have detected staphylococcus as the most common causative agent of nosocomial infections in HIV-positive patients. This is probably the result of a combination of the skin entrance of staphylococcus with the frequent use of central vascular catheters (CVCs).

Bacteraemia in HIV-positive patients is known to constitute a significant problem. CVC and urinary catheter utilisation was significantly higher among these patients in a hospital infection control study conducted by Padoveze, Trabasso and Branchini (2002: 346). These researchers also found that HIV-positive patients are more likely to have bloodstream infections than other patients. Because HIV-positive patients have high *S. aureus* carriage, they can serve as a reservoir of MRSA in hospitals and communities (Padoveze, Trabasso & Branchini 2002: 350).

Other important nosocomial infections were *Acinetobacter baumanii* and *Klebsiella pneumoniae*. Central lines are used more frequently in HIV-positive patients, which indicates that all health care workers have to be careful in using these lines.

Depletion of CD4 cells has a profound effect on the patient's immune system – as the patient is much more at risk of bacterial, fungi and other virus infections. Pathogens such as mycobacteria, salmonella, fungi and toxoplasma are pathogenic infections that play a part in life-threatening infections in HIV-positive patients. Abnormal B cell function is associated with an increased susceptibility to infections by *S. pneumoniae* and *Haemopilus influenzae*.

Furthermore, the breakdown in integrity of the skin, as a consequence of Kaposi's sarcoma and dermatoses, leads to increased susceptibility to staphylococcal and gram-negative infections. Invasive procedures and indwelling devices may be associated with bacteraemia and fungaemia. Neoplasms may be associated with a variety of organisms, such as clostridia, enterococci, *Streptococcus bovis* and gram-negative infections (Duse 1999: 193–4).

Hand-washing and disinfection should always be compulsory in any hospital or health care facility. A plastic apron should be worn in case of secretions, and a mask in case of splashes. Laundry, waste and cleaning should be done according to standard infection control precautionary measures applicable to the patient's condition. Aids patients with additional infections should be nursed in a single room and the health care workers treating them should guard against coming into contact with blood and secretions (Duse 1999: 194).

It seems possible that patients with HIV and Aids will now be able to live longer, and this will force improved infection control measures and surveillance of nosocomial infections in the future in all local health care facilities. It also seems likely that health workers will increasingly face the challenge of diagnosing and preventing these infections as the Aids pandemic progresses.

CASE STUDY

Imagine that you are a clinic nurse in charge of the antenatal clinic. You receive results from the laboratory indicating that one of your pregnant patients has XDR TB. You know that she is due to go into labour in the next week.

Question

Describe your plan of action and the infection control measures that need to be in place in this case of XDR TB.

Application to your own context

- Investigate your hospital's infection control policy regarding MDR TB and XDR TB.
- Establish the level of precautions applicable for XDR TB patients and observe if that is applied in your institution.

TIPS FOR NURSES

Always implement standard precautions as a rule and then apply precautions as per disease specifications. Wear a respirator as protection.

PRECAUTIONS

Always familiarise yourself with the infection control procedures in the health services, particularly in reference to the above-mentioned emerging diseases. Remember to apply at least the standard precautions for all patients, and ask an infection control officer if you are unsure of anything.

CONCLUSION

Clearly, MDR TB and XDR TB are mainly a human-made problem, reflecting a failure to implement the measures recommended by the WHO. These measures require political commitment and a will to improve the health of people, and if health problems are not given top priority, diseases like MDR TB and XDR TB will continue to emerge, especially in this age of HIV and Aids.

Furthermore, SARS needs continual assessment in order for rapid expansion and a health crisis to be prevented. A communication plan must be developed by all countries affected in order to prepare for a SARS pandemic. Influenza pandemics have taken us by surprise in the past. Vaccines are the most important intervention for the reduction of mortality in any country. The world has been warned in advanced about avian flu, and health care organisations and governments worldwide should plan for it. Although the avian flu virus is currently an epidemic in bird populations, the risk of the virus becoming a human pandemic is genuine.

SELF-ASSESSMENT

Before closing this book, make sure that you can discuss the following key concepts and their application in your context with a colleague:
* MDR TB and XDR TB.
* SARS.
* Avian flu.
* HIV and Aids.

FURTHER READING AND WEB RESOURCES

http://www.who.int/ tuberculosis
http://www.mrc.ac.za publications tuberculosis
http://www.cdc.gov/ncidod/EID/index.htm
http://www.slackinc.com/general/iche
http://www.his.org.uk
http://www.icna.co.uk

Conclusion

Infection control is every health care professional's business, and the Hippocratic oath informs all health care practices – health care professionals must prevent harm from coming to patients. This book adds to the knowledge of health care professionals in their everyday patient care activities in hospitals and other clinical environments. If everyone is aware of infection control, infection rates must go down.

Health care professionals are also at risk in health care settings and hospitals, where new diseases are continually emerging. Health care professionals need accessible information in order to be able to assist with infection control, as well as for their own protection against infective diseases. This book is a resource for health care professionals who are not infection control officers, but who need to practise safe health care in order to protect patients and themselves from nosocomial infections.

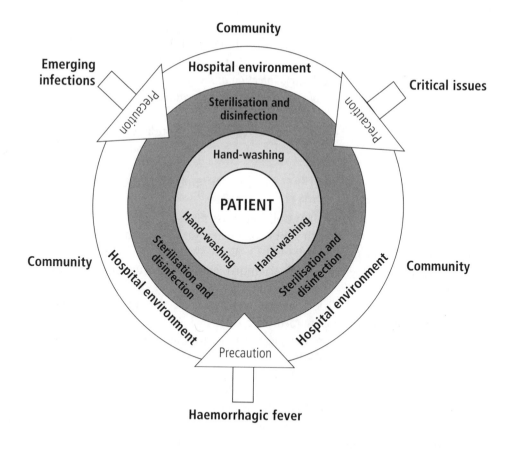

References

Barie, P. S. and Eachempati, S. R. 2005. Surgical site infections. *Surgical Clinics of North America*, 85: 1115–35.

Baron, R. M., Baron, M. J. and Perrella, M. A. 2006. Pathobiology of sepsis. *American Journal of Respiratory Cell and Molecular Biology*, 34: 129–34.

Best, M. and Neuhauser, D. 2004. Ignaz Semmelweis and the birth of infection control. *Quality and Safety in Health Care*, 13: 233–4.

Burke, P. 2007. Infection control – a problem for patient safety. *The New England Journal of Medicine*, 348(7): 651–6.

Centers of Disease Control and Prevention. 2000. Update: Outbreak of Rift Valley fever – Saudi Arabia, August–November 2000. *JAMA*, 284(23): 2989–90.

Centre of Disease Control (CDC). 2002. Guideline for hand hygiene in health-care settings. Vol 51 no RR-16 www.cdc.gov/ncidod/hip Retrieved 4 December 2006.

Cocanour, C. S., Peninger, M., Domonoske, B. D., Li, P. D. T., Wright, B., Valdivia, A. and Luther, K. M. 2006. Decreasing ventilation-associated pneumonia in a trauma ICU. *The Journal of Trauma Injury, Infection and Critical Care*, 61(1): 122–8.

Damani, N. N. 2006. *Manual of infection control procedures*. 2nd edition. Cambridge: Cambridge University Press.

Dunn, P. M. 2005. Ignaz Semmelweis (1818–1865) of Budapest and the prevention of puerperal fever. *Archives of Disease in Childhood-fever and Neonatal Edition*, 90: 245–348.

Duse, A. G. 1999. Nosocomial infections in HIV-infected/AIDS patients. *Journal of Hospital Infection*, 43: 191–201.

Duse, A. G. Infection control. Unpublished class notes.

Fisher-Hoch, S. 2005. Lessons from nosocomial viral haemorrhagic fever outbreaks. *British Medical Bulletin*, 73 and 74: 123–37.

Goad, J. A. and Nguyen, J. 2003. Hemorrhagic fever viruses. *Topical Emergency Medicine*, 25(1): 66–72.

Gupta, S. and Jonas, M. 2006. Sepsis, septic shock and multiple organ failure. *Anaesthesia and Intensive Care Medicine*, 7(5): 143–6.

Isaacson, M. 2001. Viral hemorrhagic fever hazards for travelers in Africa. *Clinical Infectious Diseases*, 33: 1707–12.

Johnson, D. R., Martin, R., Burrell, L. J., Grabsch, E. A., Kirsa, S. W., O'Keeffe, J., Mayall, B. C., Edmonds, D., Barr, W., Bolger, C., Naidoo, H. and Grayson, M.L. 2005. Efficacy of an alcohol/chlorhexidine hand hygiene program in a hospital with high rates of nosocomial methicillin-resistant *Staphylococcus aureus* (MRSA) infection. *Medical Journal of America (MJA)*, 183(10): 509–14.

Laing, R. B. S. 1999. Nosocomial infections in patients with HIV disease. *Journal of Hospital Infection*, 43: 170–85.

Larson, E. 1989. Public health then and now. *American Journal of Public Health*, 79(1): 92–9.

Lashley, F. R. 2006. Emerging infectious diseases at the beginning of the 21st century. The Online Journal of Issues in Nursing, 11(1) wwwnursingworld.org/ojin/topic29/top29-1 Retrieved 9 May 2007.

Minnaar, A. 2007. Hand-washing technique. Unpublished work.

Minnaar, A. and Bodkin, C. 2006. *The pocket guide for HIV and AIDS nursing care.* Cape Town: Juta.

Morton, P. G., Fontaine, D., Hudak, C. M. and Gallo, B. M. 2005. *Critical care nursing: A holistic approach.* 8th edition. Philadelphia: Lippincott.

Moszynski, P. 2006. Experts devise strategy to fight new TB strain. *British Medical Journal*, 333 September: 566.

Ndayimirije, N. and Kay, K. M. 2005. Marburg hemorrhagic fever in Angola – fighting fear and a lethal pathogen. *The New England Journal of Medicine*, 352(21): 2155–7.

Padoveze, M. C., Trabasso, P. and Branchini, M. L. M. 2002. Nosocomial infections among HIV-positive and HIV-negative patients in a Brazilian infections diseases unit. *American Journal of Infection Control*, 30(4): 346–50.

Pearce, J. 1997. Infection control hand-washing procedure. Unpublished work developed at the Johannesburg Hospital.

Peters, C. J., Sherrif, R. and Zaki, R. 2002. Role of the endothelium in viral hemorrhagic fevers. *Critical care medicine*, 30(5): 268–73.

Picheansathian, W. 2004. A systematic review on the effectiveness of alcohol-based solutions for hand hygiene. *International Journal of Nursing Practice*, 10: 3–9.

Ricart, M., Lorente, C., Diaz, E., Lollef, M. H. and Rello, J. 2003. Nursing adherence with evidence-based guidelines for preventing ventilator-associated pneumonia. *Critical care medicine*, 31(11): 2693–6.

Richards, G. A. 2007. Avian influenza. Unpublished work.

Richards, G. A., Murphy, S., Reeve, J., Mervyn, M., Zinman, C., Taylor, R., Swanepoel, R., Duse, A., Sharp, G., De la Rey, I. and Kassianides, C. 2000. Unexpected Ebola virus in a tertiary setting: Clinical and epidemiologic aspects. *Critical care medicine*, 28(1): 240–4.

Richmond, J. K. and Bagolbe, D. 2003. Lassa fever: Epidemiology, clinical features and social consequences. *British Medical Journal*, 327(29): 1271–5.

Rivers, E. P., McIntyre, L., Morro, P. C. and Rivers, K. 2005. Early and innovative interventions for severe sepsis and septic shock: Taking advantage of a window of opportunity. *Canadian Medical Association Journal*, 173(9): 1054–65.

Tiwari, A., Tarrant, M., Yuen, K. H., Chan, S., Kagan, S., Ching, P., Wong, A. and Wong, S. S. Y. 2006. Preparedness for influenza pandemic in Hong Kong nursing units. *Journal of Nursing Scholarship*, 38(4): 308–13.

Trautner, B. W. and Dorouiche, R. O. 2004. Catheter-associated infections. Pathogenesis affects prevention. *Arch Intern Medicine*, 164: 842–50.

Weaving, P. and Cooper, T. 2006. Infection control is everyone's business. *Nursing Management*, 12(10): 18.

Weyer, K., Van der Walt, M. and Kantor, P. 2006. Managing multi-drug-resistant tuberculosis. Legal implications. MRC Policy Brief. South Africa: MRC.

Wilson, J. and Jenner, E. A. 2007. *Infection control in clinical practice*. Edinburgh: Elsevier.

World Health Organisation (WHO). 2005. Responding to the avian influenza threat. Recommended strategic actions. who/cds/csr/gip/2005.8 Retrieved 5 July 2006.

Ziady, L. E. and Small, N. 2004. *Prevent and control infection*. Cape Town: Juta.

Zoutman, D. E. and Ford, D. 2005. The relationship between hospital infection and surveillance and control activities and antibiotic-resistant pathogen rates. *American Journal of Infection Control*, 33(1): 1–5.

Index

Please note: Page numbers in *italics* refer to tables and figures.

A
accountability 36
acid-fast bacilli (AFB) 76
Acinetobacter baumanii 78
Acinetobacter spp. 15
African haemorrhagic fevers 61, *68–69*
    precautions 70
age, extremes of 52
Aids 77–79
air, contaminated 38
airborne precautions 2, 7, 8
alcohols 17
anaemia, post-operative 53
anthrax 4
antibiotics 7
antiretroviral drug administration 77
antiseptic agents 28
    alcohol-based 17, 20
    waterless 14
antiseptic hand-rubbing 13
antiseptic hand-washing 13
anti-microbial agent 13
anti-microbial policies 5
Arenaviridae, *see* Lassa fever
Aristotle 3
ascites 47, 51
aseptic instruments 28
avian (bird) flu (*Mycobacterium avium*) 72, 73, *74–75*, 77
    preparation phases 75

B
Bacillus anthracis 19–20
bird flu, *see* avian flu
blood
    infection 55
    spills 29
    sugar control 53
    transfusion 47, 53

bloodstream infection 47
    IV device-associated 54–57
Bunyaviridae nairovirus,
    see Congo-Crimea fever
Bunyaviridae phlebovirus, *see* Rift Valley fever

C
candida 49
care managers, expectations of 22
case studies 9, 23, 30, 43, 58, 67, 79, 81–87
CD4 cell depletion 78
central sterilisation supply department
    (CSSD) 28
central vascular catheters (CVCs) 78
chemotherapy 55
chlorhexidine 4, 17–18
chloroxylenol 18
cholera 4
chronic disease 55
chronic inflammation 52
Clostridium difficile 6, 8, 15, 19–20, 77
Clostridium difficile-associated diarrhoea
    (CDAD) 40
colonic flora 49
Columbus, Christopher 4
Congo-Crimea fever (Bunyviridae nairovirus)
    61, 65
Constitution of the Republic of South Africa
    (Act 108 of 1996) 2
contact precautions 2, 8, 9
corona virus (SAR-CoV) 75
cross-infection 37
Cryptosporidium parvum 77

D
decontamination 27
    guidelines *31–33*
    of hands 13
dermatoses 78
detergent 14
diabetes mellitus 52
diarrhoea 19, 20
disease outbreak management 42–43

Disinfectant Act (1972) 13
disinfection 5, 27
    equipment and items 29–30
    precautions 33
disseminated intravascular coagulation
    (DIC) 63
drainage system guidelines 50
drop foot 3
droplet precautions 2, 8, 9

E
Ebola virus (Filoviridae filovirus)
    61, 62, 66–67
emerging infections 10, 72, 72
    precautions 79
Enterobacter cloacae 15, 49, 77
enterococcus 15, 46, 49, 51
Environmental Conservation Act
    (73 of 1989) 2
environmental factors 52–53
environmental surfaces 38
Escherichia coli 49
extremely drug-resistant (XDR TB)
    72, 76–77, 79

F
Filoviridae filovirus, *see* Ebola and
    Marburg fever
fingernails 23
flavivirus, *see* yellow fever
fluid 47

G
gloves 8, 23, 28, 29
gonorrhoea 4
Government Notice R1390 (2001) 2
gram-negative bacilli 15
gram-negative nosocomial pneumonia 77
gram-positive cocci 46, 51

H
haemodialysis water 38
Haemophilus influenzae 77, 78
haemorrhagic fever 10, 61, 62–63, 63, 72
HAI, *see* hospital-acquired infection 2
hand antisepsis 14
hand hygiene
    adherence to practices 14, 15–16
    guidelines 17–18
    specific organisms 19–20

hand-rub, alcohol-based 13
hand-washing 37
    compliance 20–21
    precautions 24
    procedures 5
    technique *21, 22*
herpes simplex 8, 17
hexachlorophene 18
Hippocrates 3
HIV 55, 72, 77–79
    transmission 73
HIV-negative patients 77
HIV-positive patients 77–78
hospital-acquired infections (HAI) 2
    see nosocomial infections
hospital environment 35, 37
    interventions 38–40
human immunodeficiency virus, *see* HIV
hygiene
    hands 15–16
    standards 7
hyperglycaemia 47, 53
hypocholesterolaemia 52
hypoglycaemia 47
hypoxemia 52

I
ileus 53–54
immune-suppressing drugs 55
immune-suppressing infections 55
infection control
    assessment guide 41–42
    critical issues 45
    history of 3–5
    model *10*
    precautions 7–9, 24, 44, 59–60
    principles 40–41
    quality control standards 6–7
infectious diseases, contributing factors 5–6
infectious spills 29
influenza 8, 38
Institute for Health Care Improvement 56
instruments 28
interferon (IFN) response 64–65
intravascular (IV) catheters
    guidelines for insertion 54
    guidelines for insertion site 54
investigations, conducting of 6
iodine 18
iodophors 18

isolation hospital, *see* lazaretto
isoniazid 73

J
Jenner, Edwin 4
jewellery 23

K
Kaposi's sarcoma 78
Klebsiella pneumoniae 49, 77, 78
Klebsiella spp. 15, 77
Koch, Robert 5

L
Lassa fever (Arenaviridae) 61, 62, 63–64
Lassa virus (LV) 63
lazaretto 2
legionella pneumophila 38
leprosy (*Mycobacterium leprae*) 4, 76
linen, contamination of 39
Lister, Joseph 4
lower respiratory tract 57

M
management
    disease outbreak 42–43
    provision of 7
Marburg fever 61, 66–67
Mastomys natalensis 63
measles 8, 38
meatus 47
medical devices, infection risks 6–7
methicillin-resistant *S. aureus* (MRSA)
    6, 15, 19, 20, 40
micro-organisms 5, 8, 48
moiety 14
multiple drug-resistant (MDR TB)
    72, 73, 76–77, 79
    seven-point plan 76
mumps 8
Mycobacterium avium, see avian flu
Mycobacterium leprae, *see* leprosy
Mycobacterium tuberculosis (M. TB) 38

N
'Naples', *see* syphilis
naso-gastric tube 57
National Health Act (61 of 2003) 2, 13,
    27, 73

National Nosocomial Infections
    Surveillance System 51
Neisseria meningitides 8
Nightingale, Florence 4
neonatal intensive care unit (ICU) 15
nosocomial infections 2, 3, 8, 10–11, 47, 57
    precautions 44
    prevention 35
    protection 10, 10–11
Nursing Act (33 of 2005) 2, 13, 27

O
obesity 52
Occupational Health and Safety Act
    (85 of 1993) 2, 13, 27
organ dysfunction 55
organisms and hand hygiene 19–20
orotracheal intubation 57
outbreak of disease 42–43

P
parenteral nutrition 54
pasteurisation 4
Pasteur, Louis 4
pathogens transmission of 14–15
peripheral vascular disease 52
personal protective equipment 28
pertussis 8
pest control 39–40
Phlebovirus, *see* Rift Valley fever
plague 4
plants and flowers contamination 39
Pneumocystis carinii pneumonia 78
pneumonia
    post-operative risk 57–58
    see also ventilator-associated pneumonia
    (VAP)
polio 3
post-operative anaemia 53
Pott's disease 3
precautions 2, 7–8, 24, 33, 44, 59–60, 70, 79
Proteus mirabilis 15
pseudomembranous colitis 19
Pseudomonas aeruginosa 18, 23
Pseudomonas infection 49, 77–78
puerperal sepsis 4

Q
quality control standards 6–7
quaternary ammonium compounds 18

R
radiation 55
research and development
    national strategy 7
resident flora 14–15
ribavirin 63, 65
rifampicin 73
Rift Valley fever (RVF) (Bunyaviridae
    phlebovirus) 61, 62, 64–65
rubella 8

S
Semmelweis, Ignaz 4, 14
sepsis 53, 55–57
    management bundle 56–57
    resuscitation bundle 56
    treatment priorities 56
severe acute respiratory syndrome
    (SARS) 72, 73, 75–76
skin of patient 15, 78
smallpox 4
soap 14, 17, 20
standard precautions 2, 7, 8
Staphylococcus aureus 8, 15, 46, 51, 77, 78
Staphylococcus epidermidis 46, 51
sterilisation 5, 27
    precautions 33
    see also disinfection
streptococcal pharyngitis 8
Streptococcus bovis 78
Streptococcus pneumoniae 78
    multi-drug-resistant 8
suction equipment 29–30
surgical hand antisepsis 14, 18
surgical mask 2, 8
surgical site infections 6, 46, 47, 49–51
    environmental factors 52–53
    patient factors 51–52
    post-operative period 53–54
    treatment factors 53
surgical stress response 53
surveillance 37
    conducting of 6
    system 2, 3, 5, 40

syphilis 4
systemic inflammatory response
    syndrome (SIRS) 55

T
TB, see tuberculosis
terminal cleaning 28
tetanus 3
tissue oxygenation impairment 52
transient flora 14
triclosan 18
tuberculosis (TB) 3, 4, 7, 8, 17, 77
typhoid 4
typhus virus, see plague

U
upper respiratory tract 47, 57
urinary catheter utilisation 78
urinary tract
    catheter-associated infections 46, 47, 48
    insertion of catheters 48
    nine-point plan 49
    prevention of infection 49

V
vaccination 4
vancomycin-resistant enterococcus (VRE) 40
Van Leewenhoek, Anton 4
varicella zoster 38
vector 2
ventilator-associated pneumonia (VAP)
    48, 57–58
    strategies for prevention 59
viral haemorrhagic fevers 63
Viridans streptococci 77

W
ward infection control checklist 83–84
waste management 39
water, contaminated 38, 77
wounds 15

Y
yellow fever (flavivirus) 62, 67